# Dying to get to Oklahoma

## Ash Mackinnon

Ash has never written a thing in his life. However he was compelled to do so after the bizarre journey he and his family were forced to endure in the hope of saving his young wife who was battling cancer. Initially, what they "discovered" by accident, which is commonplace overseas, amazed them. Yet it made them angry that we lucky Australians didn't have access to these potentially lifesaving treatments. This is part of the story. The other part of the story is the battle this family were subjected to by financial institutions and the Australian Government as a result of the costs incurred in obtaining treatment in the USA. It may not be the best written piece of work you'll read but your generosity in purchasing the book, along with information you take from it, will help others in the future. As Ash says, if this story saves one life or helps one family avoid the anguish they experienced, then it will all have been worth it.

# Inspiration

"Do your little bit of good where you are; it's those little bits of good put together that overwhelm the world."
**Desmond Tutu**

How true, mountains were not built overnight and anything worthwhile is worth waiting for. With any hope at all, I pray that as Aussies we all pull together and get this dream for you and your wife. It will be her legacy and she will always be there if her spirit can help others in this huge way!

**Marlene Williams** - Melbourne, Victoria, Australia

It feels great to know that I can help bring this product to Australia. My mother died of cancer in March 2007 & I've other relatives fighting the disease also. So really appreciate being a part of this. Thank you for the invite Ash & hope to hear more about the book when it's released. Thanking you,  Leesa

**Leesa Osmond** - Deception Bay, Queensland, Australia

You are an inspiration. Go get that book published.
**Leonie Clarke** - Sydney, NSW, Australia

I had never heard of anyone dying to get to Oklahoma. Our kids were dying to get to Disneyland when they were younger. I was dying to visit Santorini for years. A friend was dying to meet Oprah for as long as I can remember. This is our story, our journey with cancer and the unfortunate situation where a loved one was actually dying to get to Oklahoma.

# Chapter One

# Valentine's Day

It seemed like a normal weekday. But where was Leah? She was rarely out of bed before me. Where was she? It really was a bit early to be pondering such things. I had to get ready for work. I was a teacher at a TAFE college. I taught Hospitality Studies. It was the perfect job. I had great hours which really suited our family life. I worked with some great colleagues and I enjoyed the interaction with and development of the students.  So I needed to get out of bed and ready myself for work.  First up was breakfast. I was alone in the kitchen. The children weren't up as yet. Rebecca who was 7 and at primary school was still in bed. Alec, or Bim as he had been known as since he was about 4 weeks old, was now still only 18mths old and loved his sleep. He was still sound asleep as I made my breakfast.

I had my toast and a coffee. Then I hit the shower. I dressed and when I re emerged from the bathroom there was Leah and our friend Sally. Now Sally was a bit younger than us but we had taken her in as our "third" child. She worked in advertising and loved coming around and we loved having her come around. She adored the children and they just loved her. She often helped out with babysitting. Really, though, it was a bit early for Sally to be here as well. Sally was not a morning person. What was she doing around so early on a weekday morning? I didn't have time to figure this out as I had to get to work. This would be about a 45 minute trip. So I said my goodbyes and headed for the car. We had a "blueberry" coloured Ford Festiva. When I saw it I nearly died. That's what Sally was doing over so early. As it was Valentine's day, she had come over to help Leah stick pink and red love hearts all over the car. We lived on a reasonably busy road and as I approached the car people were tooting their horns at me. There must have been about 50 of those hearts all over the car. I felt so proud, so loved and the embarrassment was actually extremely enjoyable. This was a great start to the day. I ran back to give the girls and the children another kiss and tell them I loved them. Then it was off to work. I had to go via the city, Melbourne, and on to the freeway and received a lot more toots as I drove. When I stopped at traffic lights people had radiant smiles. It was amazing the impact our little blue car, with love hearts all over, had on complete strangers. Many of the hearts blew off as I drove but when I got to work and drove into the car park about three quarters still remained. I went in to work and got more ribbing and lots of oohs and aahs. This was a very memorable Valentine's day.

When I left work the hearts were still there in all their glory. I drove home getting similar reaction to the drive into work that morning. I stopped at the bottle shop on the way home to buy a bottle of champagne. I would cook dinner tonight, as I did most nights, and we could have a glass of bubbly to celebrate Valentine's day, our love for each other and for me to say thanks to Leah for being so thoughtful.

However when I arrived home it was evident that something was very wrong. Leah's mum was there. She was sobbing uncontrollably. I asked what had happened. It turned out that Leah had been to the doctor that day. She had found a lump in her breast. She had initially thought nothing of it as she had been breastfeeding until just recently. She had assumed it was a blocked milk duct or something trivial like that. However it wasn't that simple. It was cancer. I rushed to Leah. I put the champagne on the bench and gave Leah a hug. I didn't know what to say initially. I just had to be there for her. Our little world had just been rocked by the worst possible news we could ever receive. My heart sunk. It was the total opposite of how I had felt this morning. Leah was such a generous and caring person. Why had she been struck down by this illness?

We were still hugging. Leah was sobbing. I held her and asked how she was. What a stupid question. This was all new to me. It was new to all of us really. Leah explained that she had to go back for more tests but the initial findings were not good. Leah finally said she was nervous, scared and feeling sick in the stomach. It had been a few hours now since she had received the news. Her mum had been with her at the time. That was lucky as she had needed support after such news. They were both now still totally upset. Leah's mum was sad but angry. She was upset that it was Leah with this potentially life threatening illness. She said that parents weren't meant to outlive their children. It was hard to console her. But we had to focus on the positive. Leah's mum and I had shown our feelings and we had been quite self centered. This was really not about us but about Leah. We had to help Leah as best we could. We had to be strong. I felt helpless. I felt ripped off. I was sad. I actually felt quite sick. But I had to push all this aside so I could be of assistance to Leah. After all how must she be feeling? The champagne I had bought earlier that afternoon sat on the bench. It was of no use now. Valentine's day would never be the same again. After some time the initial impact of Leah's news had subsided somewhat. I made cups of tea for us all. We had to discuss this situation and how we would deal with it. Leah was still in shock and she was very scared. But we had to make plans. We decided not to tell the children just yet. I wanted to find out all the details from the doctor and get an idea of what we had ahead of us.

The next few days, waiting to get to see the oncologist, were shocking. The agony of waiting was excruciating. We had sleepless nights. We would just lie in each other's arms. We were scared. Leah was petrified. We spoke of things we had never even contemplated before in our lives. We knew nothing about the subject of cancer. This was a rapid learning experience. We cried. We didn't eat. We dropped things. We walked around in a daze. We forgot things. We had difficulty functioning with the everyday tasks of life. We had to concentrate on Leah's wellbeing above all else at the moment.

I took time off work. My employers were amazing. The staff and students I worked with were so generous and supportive. I had to be there to assist and support Leah. I couldn't juggle work, family and Leah. Leah had to be the total focus during this time. We got so much support from all areas of our lives as well. Rebecca went to a private school and people who were acquaintances at the time, now wonderful friends, all banded together to assist in any way they could. They would pick Rebecca up from school. They'd drop a box of fruit and vegetables off at the front door. Even fully cooked meals were sent over so it was one less thing we would have to worry about. One lady was a doctor and she arranged for Leah to see a fantastic oncologist. We went to see him the following week. He confirmed the worst. I had needed to hear this diagnosis for it to be real in my mind. But it was all too real. We had endured a couple of days since Leah had first received the news. Now we were going through it again. I felt sick to the stomach again. Having a professional tell me the news was extremely overwhelming. It gave the news about Leah's cancer so much more impact. She burst into tears again. I wanted to but needed to hold her, comfort her and listen to the oncologist. He set up the appointment with the surgeon who was a colleague of our friend who was also a doctor. This surgeon worked in the private sector. We didn't have private health insurance so we thought we would have to battle the public system. However private doctors are required to spend a small amount of time in the public system from time to time. We were slotted in to the schedule of this highly recommended surgeon. This was an amazing break for Leah. The learning had begun. It continued in the waiting room after this initial appointment with the oncologist.

We left the doctor's office and stopped in the waiting room to collect our thoughts. Another lady had just been given the same news as Leah had just received. This poor woman just burst into tears. As she was on her own we tried to console her and she did calm down but we just hoped she'd be okay. She was one of many who all have their own story to tell about the cancer journey. Leah had been booked in for her surgery and treatment but this lady, who was in a private health fund, had to come up with several thousand dollars before her treatment could be scheduled. This was just a sickening thought, not just for her but us as well. We couldn't help her but we stayed with her until she had settled somewhat and she was able to make some phone calls. This was one of many supportive times we would be involved in over the next number of years. Sometimes we would be fortunate enough to be able to offer support. On other occasions we gratefully accepted support from others. This was crucial in the manner cancer was dealt with.

We went home and started planning for the future. The first step had been given to us by the oncologist and Leah's surgeon. Leah required a mastectomy, many lymph nodes removed, then chemotherapy and then radiation. The initial surgery would happen the next week. The rest of the treatment would take months. I was exhausted just hearing this. How would Leah cope with actually having to go through it all? Was it all necessary? It all seemed a bit over the top. But they are the doctors and they know best right? One amazing thing about Leah is that she never even queried the urgency of having the mastectomy. Her breast didn't determine her womanhood she had said. Just do whatever it takes to get rid of the cancer and that was the attitude she had all the way through.

Leah went to hospital the next week. She underwent quite a long procedure, which started in the morning and went to the afternoon. She had been adamant that I bring the children in to visit as soon as she woke up. I waited till the kids got home from school and off we went. Now I am not overly flash where hospitals are concerned but I had to be strong. I find hospitals quite oppressive and I often become light headed when I visit them. Little did I know this was something I would have to get over very quickly as we would be spending some time in hospitals for a while. Leah was still groggy when we arrived. Doped up on some pain killers as well but a glimmer of a smile upon seeing us arrive. The kids had to be careful, no huge hugs just yet and no jumping on the bed. All in all it wasn't too bad an experience. The kids were a bit taken aback but things were going to be a bit different for a while so we had to get used to it. Leah had to stay in hospital for a few days so I would bring the children in each afternoon. Our lives remained relatively normal. I still went to work. I had taken some time off while Leah got her appointments out of the way but had returned to work when Leah had gone into hospital. Bec was at school and Bim went to his grandparents until I came home from work and it was time to visit mum each day. The day that Leah was discharged I kept the children home from school and they came in to help bring mum home (along with the massive amount of flowers, teddy bears, fruit and chocolate).

Life had now changed forever. Leah was still a bit tender after the surgery but was in great spirits and just adored being home with the family. Her parents just lived around the corner so they were an amazing help and friends dropped off everything from pre cooked food to organic fruit, books, magazines and anything to keep Leah entertained while she recovered. The feeling at this stage was of relief. The process to beat this disease had begun. It wasn't pleasant and was very invasive in many aspects of all of our lives but it was necessary and it was action that needed to be taken. But there was no time for Leah to get comfortable. She had to begin her chemotherapy. Again, it was a trek into the hospital for her regular treatments of this drug. I was amazed at the process of administering chemotherapy. The nurse would come out with a huge protective apron, the most cumbersome rubber gloves you've ever seen and safety goggles. They were putting this stuff inside a human being? But it was for the best right? It was a pretty depressing process. Lots of people, some quite young, sitting around absorbing this toxic cancer killer through intravenous tubes. Some were children. I hated it. I have no idea how Leah tolerated it. I couldn't take her each time, which I was secretly glad of, so Leah's mum took her in also. It was soon really noticeable how severe this treatment was on the body and spirit. Leah was lucky that the side effects were only minimal. Sure the hair fell out. It knocked the wind out of her sails. She was tired. She lost her appetite. But generally she could function quite normally. Even if she did need more sleep and a nana nap from time to time. Leah had the most positive and upbeat nature I had ever experienced so she coped with the process beautifully. Chemo was an interesting experience for me also. I would chat to patients and carers. All of them had very similar stories. I was amazed at the negativity though. There was not much inspiration here. Leah was determined to change that. She needed inspiration and hope. She treated it as a social occasion. She made many new friends throughout these sessions. She was determined to stay upbeat, optimistic and positive. The staff and patients loved her attitude and spunk. Leah was like a breath of fresh air for them. It must get very trying for staff dealing with people in this predicament and environment. They enjoyed having Leah around.

Our routine as a family changed as well. Being in the hospitality industry I was able to adjust how we ate and functioned for the best. We had a juicer which was rarely used previously, as I think most families would also discover, as the cleaning is a nightmare. This was now one of our most important devices. There were times Leah didn't want to eat but the juicer allowed me to provide nutrients which were essential in counteracting what the chemotherapy did to the body. We lived in a suburb that had an awesome organic grocer. Pat Wilson, the "Bop Girl" from the 80's was the proprietor and we formed a great relationship with her and she had great produce we could use in our new daily lifestyle. We all benefitted from this change, not that we ate badly, but sometimes life just takes over and you take the easy way out. We couldn't do that anymore and every part of the day was thoroughly thought through. It was expensive, cancer is expensive, but we had to put in the effort.

Chemotherapy was alright. As alright as it could be. I took over most of the household duties. I don't know how people did chemo and the daily stuff as well. We met many who were doing just that. Leah needed to concentrate on getting better. She had to leave the mundane stuff to us. After her first few sessions she began getting used to it. Sure she had the usual side effects but she was managing well. The hair had fallen out. That was hard on the kids. So she shaved it all off. Bec was devastated. She was 7 and to see mum without her long flowing blonde hair took a bit of getting used to. It was really only a few days, a week tops and it was now quite normal for the children to see mum like this. Leah could have gotten a wig but felt it uncomfortable so declined. We quickly got used to it. Leah was blessed with having a pretty head. The baldness suited her. But when we ran in to friends for the first time obviously it was still a shock. Some burst into tears. Others used humour or a compliment to deal with it. Rebecca's drop off at school was a bit difficult as well. It took a while for teachers, students and other parents to get used to it. Bec's school was a private school in Melbourne so most were quite wealthy, we were the exception, and therefore image was very important for many. But they had also been there and were still there in our time of need. They also loved our down to earth, no frills way of life and we were invited to many social functions due to these qualities. So most took Leah's new look in their stride and life just moved on.

Mrs Anderson was the head of the junior school. She reminded us of Mary Poppins and it was such a comfort to know she was looking after our child. This was the view of all the parents, at such a wonderful school. She made an announcement so everyone was on the same page and understood our situation and sent a newsletter home to ensure everyone was informed of Leah's illness. We tried to keep life as normal as possible so Leah indulged in the odd morning tea with the girls even if it meant a nap in the afternoon to recover. As time went on she needed less of a recovery as the chemo had less of an effect. She even went back to work.

# Chapter 2

# How we met

I will give you a bit of background as to how Leah and I met. At the time I had a great job at a college in Melbourne but I decided to look for a part time job a few nights per week as well. This would assist me financially and be a much needed social outlet also. I did get that job at a hotel in a seaside suburb of Melbourne. Sally, who I mentioned earlier, also worked there and that's where we met. Leah worked there to but, of course, we hadn't met yet. I worked in the cocktail bar which was part of the restaurant within the hotel. Leah worked either in the main bar or in the function room. My area was smack bang in between both of her work areas. She used to say hi to me as she went from one work area to the other. I didn't know her name so I would reply, "G'day love". This was extremely slack I know but with all the new staff at the hotel, customers and all my students at college I had so many names to remember that this was a common greeting I used at the time. I enjoyed the job immensely. It was great fun, I made great tips and it was extremely social. Then a friend of mine, Bridget, began working at the hotel also. At the time Bridget needed a place to live as well and Leah, who was house-sitting for a friend, had a spare room to offer and Bridget accepted. I still didn't know Leah that well. However I would visit Bridget on a Tuesday evening, which was Melrose Place night on the television in those days. This evolved into a regular event. I'd cook and the girls would have a chat and a laugh, then we'd all catch up with Billy, Michael, Jane and Amanda. Before long it wasn't just Melrose nights. I'd pop over during the week as well. We were all getting along really well. As a result we all decided to plan a trip to Greece. Leah had already planned a trip to visit her friend in the USA. She decided she would meet Brig and I after she had been over to the USA to catch up with her old friend. The more time it took to plan, the more I was required to go over for dinner or a cuppa and some more planning.   Then it all changed. All of a sudden Leah and I had fallen for each other. We didn't know when or how but we had. This meant our plans for the trip changed as well. So instead of Leah joining Bridget and I in Greece we were now both going to meet Brig in Santorini after Leah and I had been to the USA. The rest, as they say, is history. It changed my life. Rebecca was from Leah's first marriage and was only 1 when we met and then a few months later we were travelling the world together. I was suddenly pushing a pram around the streets of Paris, Amsterdam and Santorini. I had been married previously as well but no children. Leah and I had created an instant family.

That first trip was to set the tone of how our lives would be lived in the future. Little did we know that we would also have some other forces having a say in this journey. Life was going to be quite different from this point on. But how different, we really had no idea....

# Chapter Three

# The cancer journey continues

The cancer journey began in 2001. Leah and I had been together since 1995. It was pretty special. We weren't married. We didn't see the need to get married as we were travelling along beautifully. We had both been married before and that hadn't worked out the best for either of us. Maybe it was a case of once bitten, twice shy. We were happy with where we were in our lives at that time. We now had two children. We lived in a lovely beachside Melbourne suburb, had good income and a great lifestyle. We were also fortunate enough to have amazing friends and family. Even cancer was being dealt with easier than we had expected. I think a positive attitude makes a huge difference. Leah's attitude was sensational. I would have been a mess if it had been me who was dealing with the horrible disease. She was so positive, so up front and so pro active in her life and her treatment. There weren't many choices offered to Leah as far as her treatment was concerned. However Leah had plenty of choices on the effect the treatment would have on her wellbeing and lifestyle. It meant changes for all of us but in many cases they were changes for the better. Life's short, you don't know what the future holds, so make the most of today. That was what Leah used to say and how she would live. So this attitude and amazing support from family and friends made for some pretty interesting times. Leah actually did a stock take of her friends and she got some new and amazing ones but she also chose to let some go as well. She only wanted supportive and positive people around her. It was selfish but she had the right to be selfish during this time.

Two amazing friends she made were actually long time friends of mine and Bridget's. While Leah and Brig were living together, Anita would ring up to chat to Brig and if I was there, to me, perhaps, if she felt inclined. If Anita reads this she will laugh! Most times though we would see Leah on the phone for an hour and wonder who she was talking to. On many occasions it was Anita. They'd never met. Anita and her husband Byron lived in Tasmania. Leah and Anita hit it off immediately. There would be lots of adventures to follow. For Leah's next birthday I bought her a mystery holiday. You buy an airline ticket but you don't know the destination until you get to the airport. They are an inexpensive but exciting gift to get someone. The destination on this occasion turned out to be Launceston in Tasmania. The only people I knew in Tasmania were Anita and Byron so I rang Anita and she said she and Byron would meet us there and have dinner with us. They lived in Hobart at the time. Launceston is about 2 hours away from Hobart. We were staying at the Country Club and Casino and when we got there Anita and Byron were already there and Leah met them both for the first time. We had Rebecca with us as well and so we organised a babysitter in our room to look after her while the 4 adults, and I use the term loosely, went out for dinner. Anita and Byron had driven a couple of hours to join us. That just shows what wonderful people they are. They decided to stay the night as well to save the drive back to Hobart until the morning. Well it turned out that Leah's birthday was the same date as Byron's birthday. Byron is 10 years, to the day, older though. What an amazing start to an amazing friendship. A great night was had by all and the sore heads the next day indicated we had enjoyed a big night. Leah was not a big drinker but played her part on this occasion. I mention this night because over the years we had some amazingly happy times with Anita and Byron, some incredibly sad ones as well but the support and love from these two amazing people, for our entire family, was immeasurable and that is why they were the first and only choice as God parents for our kids. We had enjoyed our mystery holiday to Tasmania and created a wonderful friendship while we were there.

# Chapter Four

# Kicking cancers butt

The rest of 2001 was spent ensuring Leah had the best chance of beating the cancer. She had undergone numerous treatments. She was required to have a number of scans. I lost count of the number of appointments Leah was required to attend. Most of the time I had no idea what these appointments were for. She just went along and was told what to do next. It was time consuming but we also left plenty of time to ensure we enjoyed living in the moment as well. We realised very quickly how precious moments were. We had experienced some very unsavoury times while Leah was sick so we were determined to enjoy the healthy times as much as possible. Friends were even more important during these times. Catching up for a quick cuppa or inviting people over for a meal. Things we take for granted were special occasions for us all now. Family was just so dear to us during this time as well. The help we got and the joy we felt catching up with members of our extended families was such an important experience while

Leah was going through all of this. It was a shock to realise how quickly circumstances could change. Time flew by as we were so busy with work, treatments, school, kids and family. Catching up with friends and rectifying missed opportunities was a priority but it did make our lives rather hectic. It was all well worth it as our new appreciation of even the smallest things was enhanced. As the year progressed, life for Leah got so much better. The treatments had finished and her vitality was back to normal. She was experimenting with haircuts and styles and colours. She was back at work. Bec was at school and Bim at Kindergarten. My work continued, although I was no longer at the hotel as I was babysitter for the nights Leah worked. I had so much support at work and wonderful work mates who were so generous with their assistance and thoughts. Leah went back to work at the hotel a few days per week. Her job gave her some income of her own, kept her mind off things and created a great support base. The hotel owners, staff and customers were brilliant for Leah. It was like a big extended family. We would socialise outside of work hours with many of them. Work was a social time for Leah as well. It also proved to everyone that cancer wasn't getting the better of her. She would beat it. She would not let the cancer keep her down or stop her doing things in life that she wanted to.

Life was pretty much back to normal which was strange for us. It had been a while since we had experienced a normal lifestyle. Even though it was beaten, the cancer was not forgotten. We both read the book released by Jane Mcgrath with insights from her husband, Australian cricket legend Glenn. I found it really good. Leah hated it. I liked the format in which Jane described each part of her battle with breast cancer and Glenn then responded with his thoughts, involvement, concerns and insights from a partner's perspective. Leah thought Jane was too vain and focused too much on her external image. Jane had been a flight allendant and in the limelight as an international cricketers wife. Leah didn't think this was the best way to be as she felt it was more important to beat the disease at any cost. In the book Glenn commented on his frustrations, determination, uncertainty and inadequacies. I had already felt many similar emotions. I had felt, initially, as though we were being cheated. Both of us had become quite selfish at first. In Leah's case this was justified as she had to focus on getting better. My selfishness was only short lived. When I looked at Leah when she was first diagnosed I was upset for me as well as Leah. I was upset for the children. However I was also amazed at Leah's strength and her attitude. I obviously didn't like cancer and the impact it was having on Leah and our lives. I wanted my old life back. However this was not going to happen if I was thinking of myself. So I pushed these feelings aside and concentrated on what I could control at the moment and that was assisting Leah, loving her and helping the kids get through the changes in their lives as well. Reading Jane's book allowed me to gain an insight into the change of emotions we would both go through and to accept them. We would have to deal with them when they arose. It encouraged discussion between us all and that was very helpful in the way the whole family coped with all of these changes. It is a bit ironic that we would actually meet Jane and Glenn later on in our journey.

Reading, the internet and other media played a big role in our situation at the time. We knew nothing. Leah had a lot of quiet time and had not been a huge reader in the past but when you need help, guidance and information it's a great pastime to partake in. She discovered a lot during this stage of her life. Leah had become a Christian at about 20 years of age. She didn't go around preaching it but lived her life as best she could following the Christian principals. During her battle with cancer she really discovered her spiritual side and it helped her hugely and after all she could use all the help she could get. Her beliefs allowed her to have faith in what lay ahead. It gave her great comfort and enabled her to help others as well. Yes, she still had time to help others with their problems. Leah's friends and family were a great help but we are mere mortals and her Christianity gave her strength, understanding and comfort in the bad times as well as the good.

She never let the doctors give her a prognosis or she never asked things such as "how long have I got?" Leah's attitude was that doctors are only human and can't really know such things. She had also heard a number of stories where the mind played a huge part in recovery or actually the demise of patients suffering from cancer. We met a family who told us of their husband / father. He had been given 6 months to live. He died on the exact day he was told he would die. Leah didn't want the doctors to give her such information. So she decided not to encourage such thoughts of an expiry date. We actually met another young lady in the waiting room one afternoon. She was on her own, drinking custard out of a carton as her throat was so sore as a result of the cancer treatment she was on. We asked her if she had any support, anyone to assist her at the doctors. She was married but her husband worked long hours and he was tired upon getting home from work. This meant she was left to attend all of her appointments alone, look after the kids and do the meals and household chores. But she explained to us that he was taking two weeks off in six months time. This was the time when the doctors had said she was expected to die! Her husband was taking time off to be with her at this time and to help with the funeral arrangements. We were devastated by this story but each person's journey is different. We tried to talk her into fighting it and changing attitudes but she worshipped her doctor and his word was gospel. She was filling in time. That experience really affected both Leah and myself. A dear old friend told Leah this young lady was sitting in God's waiting room. We hated cancer.

# Chapter Five

# Patrick Swayze and here we go again

Anita and Byron, who I spoke of earlier, asked us if we wanted to travel on a big trip with them. Well who wouldn't? We didn't need to be asked twice. We all got on so well and Anita and Byron didn't have kids of their own but just adored Rebecca. We didn't have Bim at this stage of our lives. So we organised a trip. This all happened a few years before Leah's cancer but is important to this story. We arranged an Amtrak train tour of USA and a side trip to Mexico. We only had Rebecca at the time so the five of us took off on an adventure. Highlights included Disneyland, New York City, Savannah on the day that Princess Diana died, Memphis and New Orleans. We finished up in Cancun and Cozumel in Mexico. The train was an awesome way to travel. Rather than hopping from point A to point B we got to see all the sights in between. We met so many people as well as we mingled with others in the carriages on the train as we went.

Part of this trip involved a visit to Universal studios in Los Angeles. We had a look around, did the tourist rides and then decided to indulge in some margaritas and nachos at the Hard Rock cafe. We liked the Hard Rock and always visited one if there was one in a city we were visiting. When we finished our food and drinks we went to leave but a velvet rope prevented us from doing so. Security guards were everywhere. They said we couldn't stand at the exit, which was where we were stalled at the time, due to the crowds. We used Rebecca, in her pram, as an excuse for not being able to move. We also used the excuse of not being able to understand the American accent of the frantic security guards who were trying to usher people away from the area where we were standing. It all seemed to work because we stayed in that spot until we worked out what was going on. The reason for the unusual activity was the 20th anniversary celebrations of Dirty Dancing the movie and Patrick Swayze was attending. Everyone was meant to be on the other side of the red carpet and the ropes. But we stood firm and Patrick and his gorgeous wife came past us on the way to the cinema where the presentation of Dirty Dancing was being shown. We yelled out, or should I say Leah screamed out, as everyone else was. But we had one advantage. We were from Australia and on the wrong side of the rope from all the other fans. Leah yelled "Hi Patrick we've come all the way from Australia" and he turned and said hi and waved. It was a highlight and little did we know Patrick would feature in our lives again at a later stage and under much different circumstances. We still talk about that day with great fondness as Leah's boldness had created an amazingly memorable moment.

We continued on our tour of the USA after that highlight. We loved the trip. New York City was everything we thought it would be. It was vibrant, multi cultural and enthralling. We likened it to Melbourne but bigger. Savannah was glorious. We arrived to the news Princess

Diana had been killed in an accident. The locals thought we were British and were very sympathetic. We were all quite stunned and we thanked the locals for their kind wishes. We visited Memphis and all that is Elvis and the blues. Elvis would also feature more in our lives in the future. We stopped in New Orleans. We stayed in the French Quarter and another lifelong dream had been fulfilled. Then we went down to Mexico to relax and take in some different culture. This was an extremely valuable and memorable trip. But I really need to get back to the cancer story.

Life with Leah's cancer had settled into some sort of routine and was, at times, somewhat mundane. Others would hate that. We loved it as it meant no cancer dramas. Leah still had her regular checkups. But she wasn't having any treatments. There were no drugs required to counteract the side effects of any cancer treatments. Leah had gone many months now and had been all clear, which was amazing. Her hair had grown and she had so much more energy and enthusiasm which made life for the whole family so much more enjoyable and rewarding. Then it happened. Leah went for her regular check up and our worst fears were realised again. The cancer was back. Due to the regularity of Leah's checkups it was caught early. The cancer was in the other breast and a few other spots this time. Catching it early was a good thing. We heard nothing negative from anyone. Doctors, the oncologist and other staff said it should be easily treated as it was caught straight away. The treatment plan would be less invasive this time. Leah only needed a lumpectomy and then back on the chemotherapy and radiation. With all the tests and treatments Leah had received in the past, she found it difficult to take the intravenous dosage of the chemotherapy this time. The doctors and nurses had trouble finding a suitable vein to administer the drug. It would take quite a lot of searching and would result in Leah coming home black and blue from bruising. It was just another inconvenience Leah had to endure. Most people hate getting needles at the best of times but to have staff try and try again was so painful, upsetting and frustrating for Leah and infuriating for me to witness. We needed a solution for this predicament. We mentioned this to Leah's oncologist and it was suggested that a porta cath be installed to make it easier for all concerned. The porta cath was a little plug inserted through an operation into the area just below Leah's collarbone. This would stay in permanently and allow staff to insert the intravenous needle into this plug each time she needed any internal drugs or treatment. This was done, treatment began and as we were old hands at it, the process was amazingly easy this time as we just slipped into cancer mode. A few different opportunities presented themselves this time around. We were much more aware and educated about the situation on this occasion. So we felt we had more control.

Leah had been reading and networking and had read an inspirational story about Dr Ian Gawler. Ian was a veterinarian surgeon and about 20 years previously was diagnosed with cancer and given six months to live. There you go. This was another reason not to let the doctors guess your future. Ian is still going strong today. But given such a prognosis, he was sparked into action. He travelled to places like India and the Philippines and sought faith healers and spiritual guru's. He learnt from dieticians and doctors. He consulted herbalists and naturopaths. He attended sessions with yoga teachers and meditation experts. He brought all of this experience and knowledge together, with various willing practitioners, to form a retreat called the Gawler Foundation retreat. It was a live in retreat. Fully catered with an emphasis on healing the body, mind and the spirit while ridding yourself of hideous disease and nurturing yourself back to health. Leah read about this, enquired and was so keen to go that she almost jumped out of her skin. But it was expensive. We had lost a lot of income in the previous two years and paid out so much in expenses such as scans, medication and supplements. But after chatting to people at her work a few of them decided to put together a fundraiser. It was an amazing concept. Friends and strangers donated items to be auctioned at a function on a lazy Sunday afternoon. However it grew way beyond Leah's expectations. A couple of hundred people turned up and the hotel supplied some drinks and food and the venue and a great event took place. The generosity of all the people involved was unimaginable. People we knew and loved, along with strangers or acquaintances, just unleashed an afternoon of giving and helping. The feeling in the room was just so uplifting and positive. The strangers became friends. People created friendships. Everyone had gathered together on this special afternoon for a united cause and Leah was not the only one to benefit. Hundreds of photos were taken as special moments, which would live in so many people's memories, were created. Everyone had a great time. There was a band and a few hours of auctions and people caught up with friends they normally wouldn't have had the time to catch up with. Our family's, from far and wide, got together. Leah's cancer had created a few really forgettable memories but it also left many with lifelong and life changing episodes. The items for auction were quite varied. Football jumpers. Club memberships. Lobsters and other delicacies. One of a kind works of art. Wine and Champagne. People donated what they could to help. In the end it was Leah everyone had turned up for and to help with her desire to be able to attend the Gawler retreat at the Yarra Valley. The auction allowed this to happen. Enough money was donated to allow Leah to go. So we started planning.


It was a live in retreat and Leah would be away for ten days. Even in hospital she had never been separated from us, predominately the children, for more than a night. In hospital we were able to visit and then she was home in the blink of an eye. The Gawler retreat was set up as an intense ten days of self reflection, indulgence, and development. No visitors. Although at meal time she would be allowed to telephone us. No mobile phones or other electronic devices were allowed so Leah would have to use the office phone which was made available for this purpose. As there would be other residents also requiring the phone it would be a quick five minute catch up. We booked Leah in. These little victories were so important to Leah's wellbeing. She was so fortunate throughout her journey to be able to have access to things we wouldn't normally be able to access. We ate a lot of organic food that a friend actually stocked in her shop in Elwood. Leah's boss at the hotel was a supplier of a range of expensive supplements which helped Leah's body after the rigours of chemotherapy and radiation. We had access to amazing doctors and surgeons and now, Dr Ian Gawler. This made her battle a lot bit more tolerable and again it was winnable.

Leah packed her suitcase and I gathered the children and we drove Leah to her retreat. It took about 90 minutes. We stopped at Warburton, a quaint little country town, on the way and had a break at a lovely organic bakery. We had deliberately tried to turn this trip into a treat for the children. They were not overly happy about mum being away for ten days. Everything we did along this cancer journey had little surprises for the children. They needed these treats to remain strong. They had been required to endure a lot of things young kids shouldn't be subjected to. A trip to the hospital would result in something trivial such as a balloon or if Leah was not feeling well at home I would take the children out of the house for a little outing. This was a long car ride for us all so a pit stop at a nice bakery was the order of the day. After our break in Warburton we continued on to drop Leah at her destination. The retreat was glorious. We were able to have a quick look around this peaceful, idyllic venue. It had beautiful, natural surroundings. The grounds contained kangaroos, parrots, kookaburras and other wildlife. The serenity was noticeable. It was perfect. We didn't want to prolong this part too long so we helped Leah with her bags, had a quick wander about and then said our goodbyes. This was extremely difficult. But it had to be done. After a very difficult and emotional goodbye I bundled the children in to the car and away we went. I must say that Bec and Bim put up with so much and still do today but have been utterly amazing in all aspects of the scary journey that they were also such a big part of.

Leah was away for the ten days but experienced life changing activities, food and people. At the beginning of her stay the staff assessed each participant individually and devised a diet and menu  to suit the persons stage of cancer, type of cancer, body type and the like. Leah was put on to thirty days of raw food and juices. Sounds yucky but they were so good at making this organic and nutritious food taste amazing. I actually bought the cookbook so I could continue the specialist diet upon Leah's return. Activities included laughter therapy and poetry. They did drawing. Painting and writing. They wrote their own eulogy. Death was broken down, scrutinised, laughed at and made less scary. It is a part of life after all. They celebrated the past, present and future. They did yoga and meditation. They met with psychologists and naturopaths. The participants had sessions with doctors and acupuncturists. They could access vitamin c therapy if this was suitable. This is huge doses of vitamin c, which, as a water soluble vitamin, causes a cleansing effect of the body. They looked at lifestyle and environment. Presenters explained about our exposure to all the unnatural foods and beverages we consume and the effect this can have on us. Even the containers for our food can be hazardous. Leah had always liked to drink water each day but she was urged to look at what type of container it was stored in. Plastic is not the best. Leah also discovered about her body and what was best for her. We quite often make inappropriate food choices for our body types. The sessions covered subjects such as food combining, allergy testing, blood types and similar topics. Leah wrote reams of notes. She came home with a library of books. She also had created a support network of people and professionals she could and would utilise in the future on a regular basis.

While she was away, Leah rang every night and let us know what they were having for dinner. She quickly filled us in on what they had experienced during the day, who her roommates were and the activities she had been a part of. We were in awe. It was such a packed schedule but was also relaxing and mind opening. She was absolutely blown away by the experience. She had allowed us to share the experience with her even though she was so far away. Her vitality fuelled our excitement as well. We were caught up in our day to day life of school, work, meals and the like so we looked forward to our phone call each night and the ten days flew by. It was good that we were busy as it made it appear like the time was going by quickly and we were less aware of how much we missed Leah. Soon it was time to pick Leah up. I bundled the children into the car and off we went again. This time, when we arrived, we were able to go in, spend some time at the retreat, help mum with her bags, meet the staff and all the other participants. They were lovely, lovely people who had been looking forward to meeting us as Leah had talked nonstop about us throughout her stay. We saw the round room where yoga and meditation took place. We went out and hugged the tree Leah had hugged every day. We saw the vegetable garden and the herb garden. We said our goodbyes and thankyous. Then we packed the car. Leah said her own sad but fond farewell and off we went. The Gawler retreat is in the Yarra Valley and close to Mt Donna Buang. Leah didn't want to go straight home after such an experience. We decided to drive up and spend some time in the snow up there. It's only about 10 cm deep at most but the children were still young enough to find this exciting. Leah was right. This was a nice way to get together again as a family.

We then drove home to start another new phase in our lives. This new life included some techniques, picked up at the Gawler retreat, that both of us would include in our lives. Leah had done a lot of meditation and I decided to get involved in this and other self improvement activities that Leah brought back with her. She had met a wonderful, gentle man by the name of Bob Sharples at the Gawler retreat. Bob is a wise man who offers meditation classes. Leah had brought back one of his cassette tapes which I still use today. It had one guided meditation track called the temple of silence which is an amazing experience and got me into meditation for the first time. Other inspirational teachers and authors Leah had discovered at Gawler were Louise Hay, Deepak Chopra, The Dalai Lama and Ekhart Tolle. This new knowledge and understanding allowed Leah to remain focused and strong in the face of such adversity over the years. It was also a wonderful and eye opening experience for me. Louise Hay has a morning and evening meditation, which can be done in bed. I still use this today.

# Chapter Six

# Elvis and a honeymoon for six

Having Leah away from home for such a long period of time made me realise a number of things. I had been able to use the time apart to reflect on events and circumstances we were currently faced with. We had both been married before and were both adamant that we had the perfect situation now and marriage was not a necessity to prove our love for each other. However I put myself in Leah's shoes and tried to envisage the feelings she would have had going through this battle with cancer. Outwardly she displayed a demeanor of calm, positivity and optimism. Friends, family or strangers picked up on these attributes and were amazed at her attitude while faced with such an awful situation. I had seen her at her lowest though. I had been with Leah behind closed doors. I had seen her not able to move. I had left her to sleep for hours and taken the dog for a walk so she could have peace and quiet. I had cleaned up vomit due to the reaction to the chemotherapy. I had slept on the couch as Leah was too hot and I would have made it worse. I had rubbed ointment into her scalp or her feet if she had a rash or dry skin. I didn't think twice. It had to be done. I would have preferred not to have needed to do it. But during these times we didn't have a choice. I am grateful that these really bad times were few. Leah generally handled her cancer treatments very well. It could not have been easy facing such uncertainty during this phase of her life. I was with her to support her. We had met others in similar situations and the partners had been either totally supportive as well or, on the other hand, couldn't cope or that perhaps broke up the relationship. We had seen the latter a couple of times and even though Leah never commented on it personally, I could imagine it would be a scary thought in the back of her mind. She used to comment to me on why I bothered to stick around. It upset me as thoughts of leaving had never entered my mind. The cancer was just a thing we had to deal with at the time. During this time I looked at where we were and what would be best for us. What would be best for Leah? We were in love and had two brilliant children and for me the natural progression at this stage of our relationship was to get married. I wanted to show my support, commitment and strength. I wanted to give Leah the reassurance of my love for her and for her own sense of security for the future. So to confirm all of this I arranged a dinner at a restaurant by the bay in Melbourne. I told her it was just a night out to take our minds off things, change of routine and spoil ourselves. We dressed up and went out to dinner. By ourselves. We had a lovely evening, laughing and doing things, together, that we hadn't had a chance to do much lately. After main course I handed Leah a card and in it I had written a note. Will you marry me? We both burst into tears. She was overjoyed. This was a truly special night. The waiter sent over a couple of glasses of champagne. We had been ready to go home but ended up staying for ages more as we had a renewed energy. Adrenalin, nerves and excitement had taken over. It was such a magical night. This was another life long memory created by this hideous disease called cancer. This was one of the good ones though.

The upcoming wedding was a great time for Leah. She could spend time planning the wedding which would take her mind off other factors in her life. She was in good health at present. She had done her chemotherapy and more radiation. She had been away to the Gawler retreat. The wedding was a chance to focus on positives, leave the cancer behind her and move into the future. She was able to do girly things with friends rather than feeling less than feminine with her bald head and scars. One thing that became apparent for Leah was the cost of a wedding these days. Things had changed since the first time we had both been in the position of arranging a wedding. I told her not to worry but she felt it was a waste of money as we had spent so much on things associated with her cancer treatment. Having cancer is an expensive part of life. Leah was periodically having scans. She was off work for periods at a time so she suffered loss of wages. There are many more incidentals that you don't even think about that cut into a family budget. At such a happy time these factors upset Leah. I joked about eloping as a cheaper way of doing it and she actually liked the idea. She thought it would be such a romantic way to get married. She researched it all. Firstly Leah looked for places we could go to elope. The Whitsundays, Bali, Thailand and even Scotland were places that appealed. Then we found the ideal place. For a fraction of the price of a traditional wedding at home we decided to go to Las Vegas for an Elvis wedding in a chapel and then go on a trip for our honeymoon. We could arrange it all on the internet. We saw the chapels on each of the wedding sites. We were able to watch videos of other Elvis weddings. We could see the schedule to see times that we could fit into. There was also a table with the costs and legalities of it all. It was exciting, unique and very easy to arrange. We invited everyone that we were going to invite to our traditional wedding at home. However due to the cost and time involved many wouldn't be able to attend. So in the end only 12 of our friends could come. We were fine with that. This wedding was for Leah. It took months to arrange and the actual event would last for over a month as well. This was a refreshing time for Leah. The wedding had the added bonus of showing Leah a secure future. Even if no one could attend we would do it as a family. We were so lucky that a dozen friends had decided to join us. Others wouldn't miss out either. They would be able to watch from home via the webcam in the chapel. This was a perfect solution and something quite unique.

Pete, my best mate and best man at my first wedding was coming and would be best man again. Pete's a top man. He took time out of a very busy schedule to attend. Pete runs a ski lodge in Methven in New Zealand. His partner and her 3 girls also came. Pauline, a jeweler who was creating our rings and who was Leah's friend from childhood would also come. Pauline was bringing her daughter, Tess, whose dad lived in the USA anyway. Pauline's partner would meet us in Europe later. Leah had a friend in San Diego, who had lived in Melbourne during their high school days, so she and a friend would come as well. I had met Kelene when Leah and I had first travelled to the USA just months after we had met. Kelene, who was from the USA, had attended school in Melbourne with Leah many years prior. Kelene's dad had designed the spire which sits on top of the Melbourne Arts Centre and he was required to come to Melbourne for a time during its design. I had met Kelene a couple of times and this would be a sensational way to catch up again. As we had so many children between us all, we decided to fly in to Los Angeles and go to Disneyland first. This would be the perfect start to the entire experience. This was going to be a great experience for our 2 children as well. They had put up with so many changes in the past couple of years. This would be an awesome treat for them. However I secretly think the adults enjoyed it more as a treat than the kids did. We had an amazing few days in Anaheim. It reminded Leah and I of our first trip away many years prior. It was great for Bim to experience the wonder which is Disneyland. Bec had already been to Disneyland before but was quite young on that first trip. She enjoyed having Tess around who was about the same age. This was also a great opportunity to catch up with friends. Pete lived in New Zealand so prior to the wedding it was really nice to catch up with a lifelong buddy in such a relaxed atmosphere. Warm days at Disneyland were followed by casual drinks and a get together for dinner. After our time at Disneyland we had Mickey Mouse ears, a life time of memories and dozens of photos. The kids all slept so well at night after the days riding the Matterhorn, Splash Mountain and the Tea Cups. This experience was a magical distraction from our usual routine revolving around cancer. It took just a couple of days to relegate cancer to a distant memory. After an amazing time at Disneyland we flew to Las Vegas. We were staying at the Hard Rock Hotel and Casino. We liked the Hard Rock. When we had travelled previously we had discovered the merits of the Hard Rock around the world. We could always get a cheapish meal there. The kids were well looked after. We like the Hard Rock memorabilia which enabled us to get an individual and unique souvenir from whichever city we were in at the time. We usually chose things which were easy to pack and transport whilst we were on our travels. Things like a T-shirt or a shot glass were the norm. We also knew the standard of these venues around the world which meant we could book in confidence. It's not the most exotic food but old favourites were the same all around the world. So the Hard Rock seemed perfect. The fact that this one in Vegas was also a hotel was a bonus. It was huge. It had a massive casino attached to it. Pete, Wendy and the girls stayed at the Hard Rock as well. Pauline was a single mum which meant her budget was a bit tight so she had booked another hotel. We went to drop her at her hotel on our way past. However when we arrived it was way too seedy. We couldn't let her stay in such a place. This was a celebration. Leah said that

Pauline and Tess would stay with us. Our room was massive. It had two king size beds so Pauline, Tess and Bec would be in one bed and Bim, Leah and I in the other. Problem solved. It worked out brilliantly. Not cramped at all.

We still had some wedding plans to arrange. We needed a marriage license before the wedding could proceed. To get a marriage license we had to go to the Vegas courthouse which was Downtown and not near the Strip where we were staying. Going to get the license was an adventure in itself. We made a day of it. It actually made a refreshing change from all the glitz of the Strip. This holiday was so good for Leah. She was happy and excited. Her past illnesses seemed like a distant memory. We all loved it. Leah had bought a lovely sky blue satin dress for her wedding gown and I had found a lovely single breasted, satin lapelled dinner suit at an op shop in Melbourne. I just needed the pink ruffled shirt to finish off the outfit and we found one at a party hire place on the way back from obtaining the marriage license. Getting the license was an interesting experience. The court was in the business area of Vegas which was totally different to the busy casino area. People were going about normal business life in this area. The courthouse was like any other court in the world. Criminals, police and witnesses were lining up to get in to the building and be part of proceedings inside. We had to join the queue. Others seeking a marriage license were also with us in the line. It was quite an interesting feeling. We were lining up with people who had committed crimes and were going into the building through a different door to us. After a while in the line we entered the courthouse, filled out the appropriate forms and received our marriage license. Our time at court was a lot less than many of the others who had appointments to keep with the judge. That left us plenty of time for lunch in one of the downtown diners. This was an awesome experience in itself. We were waited on by the true American diner waitress. She offered tuna salads and burgers. We drank malted milk shakes and sodas. It was like being part of a Hollywood movie.

That night we were in for another huge surprise. Pete took us to an exceptional restaurant for our pre wedding dinner. Nobu must be one of the world's most spectacular restaurants and we were there. All thanks to my buddy Pete. I was embarrassed by the generosity of the man but as I had experienced with Anita and Byron, Leah's parents, Pete so many times and complete strangers, people cared. They wanted the best for Leah. This was another overwhelming experience for everyone there but also one that would remain in my memory for ever. Leah had tackled cancer numerous times and the support she had received during these times was quite amazing. People offered things such as time, money, past experiences, support or the sharing of emotions. Whatever people could afford was offered and made us all feel quite humble. It still does, reflecting upon this journey. It all added to the experience. We had experienced amazing times even during some really bad times. Now we were in the middle of such a huge adventure from what started as a simple marriage proposal. We all enjoyed this once in a lifetime dinner at Nobu on the eve of our most special day. Pete had done it again. He had done it in such a big way. Dinner was amazing. It was the perfect experience to lead us into our big day. The next day we would be married. But a lot can happen in a few hours. That night Bim, who was asleep in the bed with us, flung his arm around in his sleep and hit Leah in the eye with his hand. She woke in such a fright but went back to sleep. However in the morning she woke with a black eye. It was so funny in a bizarre way. When we were all awake and realised what had happened, we rolled around laughing. We had most of the day to get ready for the wedding and Leah was able to apply sufficient make up to cover the bruising and the wedding went ahead as planned. This was something you only see in movies. But the girls were able to perform a miracle. Leah looked beautiful in her sky blue dress she had bought in Australia and brought with her for the occasion. Bec wore a Rapunzel style dress that made her look like a princess. It was brilliant having the children, or as Elvis said, our hound dogs, with us. Kelene, our friend from San Diego, was a great help with baby minding duties, with Bim, as he was only about three. She also videotaped most of the wedding. I had heard about a female's ability to multi task.

The chapel was amazing. It was very Vegas but also very Hollywood. We were ushered in by the coordinator in charge. We had a quick rehearsal with a staff member and then it was time. We assumed our positions and Elvis entered the building. He was a young, slim Elvis. Love me tender, Viva Las Vegas and a few other songs were performed. There was dancing, during the wedding, which I had never experienced before.  A few lines of marriage vows from Elvis and before you knew it we were married. We had lots of dancing again after we were pronounced husband and wife. Then it was time for lots of photos and good times followed. A celebrant sealed the deal in a room adjacent to the chapel to make it legally binding. As we left the chapel, a huge stretch Hummer limousine greeted us. Pete had arranged this as a surprise. I told you he is a top man. I have known Pete for thirty years and I cannot begin to describe the support he has offered. This man had been there side by side with me in many great times but a few not so good times as well. As a man I could not ask for a better best buddy, albeit from afar in the last decade or so. So in this glorious Hummer limo and before we headed to the reception we were given an awesome tour of the famous Vegas Strip at night with all the lights and mayhem it's so famous for. We cruised past Bellagio's casino and the dancing fountains, the Pirate show, the fake Eiffel tower and the amazing opulence of the Vegas Strip. Then we headed off to the Hard Rock Cafe for the reception. We walked in and there was dancing on the bar. Music was playing, bar staff tossing bottles around while mixing cocktails and waiters frantically taking food and drinks out to the many tables. This was a great choice for the reception as there was something for everyone. One of the booths had a framed picture of the Rat Pack above it so we used that as a prop for some great photo's. We loved Dean Martin so this was a fitting end to this amazing day. We ate basic food such as burgers, chicken strips, sundaes and fries but there was something for everyone. It wasn't about the food as such but more about the day. We had done it. We were married. We let our hair down and enjoyed the night. It may have been quite basic but it was definitely a night to remember. That night we rang Leah's parents to share the news. They were very happy for us and would catch up with it all when we returned to Australia and showed the video.


Next though was the honeymoon. We woke up the day after the wedding and decided to have a relaxing day at the resort. We would just laze by the pool. A few drinks, the kids could swim and we could just enjoy the time together. It was Spring so quite warm. It really was great weather for swimming and not doing much else. Later that night Kelene and her friend said goodbye and returned home. They had enjoyed the experience and it was nice for Kelene to have enjoyed Leah's special day. The next day Pete and his partner and the girls also went back home to New Zealand. As you can imagine, I couldn't thank Pete enough. Just to have him at our wedding was enough. But he had done so much more and really made it special. Later on that day Pauline, Tess and our new family set off for Germany and the start of our honeymoon. We still laugh at the fact that Pauline spent our wedding night in our hotel room with us and then came along on the honeymoon. Great memories and we wouldn't have had it any other way.

We flew from the USA to Frankfurt in Germany. We met up with Pauline's partner at this time. Then, after a few days in a number of stunning different villages, we caught the train along the Rhine River to Amsterdam. This was an awesome trip. The scenery was breathtaking. The train was certainly a brilliant way to travel. Leah's family, on her mother's side, was Dutch and Leah had lived in Amsterdam for a year when she was 18 years old. We had a week in Amsterdam and Leah showed us around. It is an amazing place. Leah showed us the tulips, the coffee shops, the canal tours and the markets. We ate veal croquettes and frits with mayonnaise. We visited galleries and historic sites. We really enjoyed our time in Amsterdam. Next it was off to Paris. It really is the city of love. What an awesome place to spend a significant part of your honeymoon. We stayed at a funny little private hotel called Hotel Comminnes. This hotel was run by Chinese but was the French Fawlty Towers. The children still love talking about our time in Paris. They still tell stories of Hotel Comminnes, especially dad sitting on a chair and it breaking under him. Or what it was like going to the shared toilet in the hall, locking the door and still being able to see and be seen through the 1 cm gap in the door. It had a lot of character and the owners were funny characters themselves. So we ended up in Paris for our honeymoon, who wouldn't want that? We climbed The Eiffel Tower, took in the views, kissed and cuddled and got the best honeymoon photos. The Louvre on Good Friday was amazing as in Australia most things are closed. We got to see some of the most stunning artwork hanging and displayed in this gallery, many of which had quite strong religious images and quite spectacular given the time of year. Later that night we went to the Moulin Rouge, although just from the outside as we couldn't afford the cost of going and seeing the show. So we ate dinner in a cute little French bistro across the road. During the days we wandered through shops and sampled French perfume. We ate crepes from street vendors. We gazed in patisserie windows. We bought baguettes and cheese and sat in the park to eat. It was a lovely romantic time. Even with Pauline, Neil and the children with us all the way. It was actually good having Pauline and Neil with us because we could take it in turns to baby sit and give each other a night to spend on our own. From Paris we went, by train, to the South of France and enjoyed the country side. We visited Arles, where Van Gogh did a lot of his work and the fortified towns in that region. The history here was amazing and the pace was certainly a lot slower than in Paris. We loved the little villages in this part of the world. We saw landmarks we had seen before in our lives in paintings or movies. After really enjoying this region we travelled over to Italy where we stayed at Portofino which was just stunning and we absolutely loved the feel of the place and the surrounding towns. Portofino is the playground of the rich and famous and we were there. We walked everywhere in Portofino. We strolled along paths that millions would have walked previously over the years. The seaside was brilliant. This area had something for everyone. Lovely little cafes, the best gelato you could imagine and sheltered beaches and parks for the children. We then travelled to Spain and spent time on the coast and went to Valencia and Barcelona. We loved Spain. It has so much history and the architecture is so varied. We would travel down little lanes and come across an amazing church or a market that had locals buying and selling local produce. We enjoyed our time so much and because of this it features again in another part of our lives in a future chapter of this story. Soon, though, our trip was over. An amazing trip filled with glorious memories and enjoyed with wonderful friends.

We returned, after our honeymoon, to life as usual. It was our old life. However cancer was now a distant memory. You will notice that I have written the word cancer throughout this story with a small "C". Leah had said not to write cancer with a big "C". Writing cancer with a small "C" diminishes its power. This makes it smaller and less powerful than if you write it powerfully with a capital. I was happy to do anything to try and diminish the power of the word. This would make it appear smaller and less threatening. Leah was so precise in her quest to beat the rotten disease. When we returned home Leah was fine and we had turned a corner so it was onward and upward with our new married life. I returned to the same job, so did

Leah. The children went back to their same school and kindergarten. We caught up with our friends and family as we used to do. We all had the same problems and the same commitments. Life was good but we had experienced so much and wanted to experience more. Feeling like this got us both thinking about the future quite differently. We were both about to make a number of interesting decisions. I will share mine first.

## Chapter Seven

# The snip and the party

Our lives were quite blissful at that moment. Leah still had to go for her regular checkups but they kept coming back with great results so we kept feeding off the positivity. Leah had been through the wringer over the last few years but we felt like we had turned a corner. The wedding and the honeymoon had helped Leah amazingly. The cancer had become a distant memory. We had come back from the wedding refreshed and determined to look positively toward the future. We had done so much to get on top of the cancer and turn our lives around. Leah had done most of it. I was just along for the scary ride. But I felt that there was much more that I could do. I actually felt that there was more that I should do. She deserved it. Leah had done most of the hard stuff. Now that she was better and we were married we were both so much more relaxed. We were able to put some time into our relationship again. What we had been through plays havoc with a relationship. Our intimacy returned to what we felt was normal. Because of this Leah decided to go back on the contraceptive pill. Then it hit me like a ton of bricks. We had two great children but another now was not in our plans. Leah had been through so much previously. Her body had been through more. Pregnancy was not even a consideration. However I was also worried about more chemicals buzzing around in Leah's body. Not to mention the hormone changes due to this. So I decided that this was my opportunity to do something to prevent Leah from having to take the pill. I told her I wanted to have a vasectomy. This was the best preventative action we could take. It was my time to go under the knife. This would be my supreme sacrifice. It was time to give her body a break. This was the natural thing for me to do. It was a natural progression for me to step up and have my "major surgery" to enable us to move forward without any unnecessary drugs. Maybe they would give me a little anesthetic prior to the dreaded snip!

Now a little snip under local anesthetic was trivial compared to what Leah had been through so far. But it was still daunting for me. I used to look at Leah in awe when I considered what she had endured and the manner in which she accepted it and then moved on during her various cancer treatments. If it were me I don't know how I would have coped. I think I would have given up ages ago. I am sure that is why I was so determined to assist Leah in any way I could. We set the vasectomy wheels in motion. Leah went to her oncologist for a checkup and I tagged along. The oncologist's office was in a suite with other medical professionals so he was able to arrange an appointment with a colleague for my vasectomy. It would be done on the Friday afternoon. This would allow me the weekend to recover. I went in after work, sat in a reclining medical lounge and the doctor performed the procedure. It was fairly straight forward, reasonably quick and without much pain. Not much pain at the time anyway. Leah was waiting for me and drove me home from the doctors, which was a role reversal for us. I was told there could be a bit of swelling and a bit of discomfort and I should get the frozen peas from the freezer and settle in for a TV marathon with little physical exertion. Again the roles were reversed and Leah had her patient to look after for the weekend. The recovery allowed me to indulge in watching a couple of games of football on television and eat soup and toast on the couch. I had two days of discomfort compared to months of traumatic procedures endured by Leah over her time with cancer. You could hardly compare the two situations but this was a small way in which I could again show my commitment to our relationship. The next week I went back to work but I felt quite proud of the sacrifice I had made. I had done this to ensure Leah had as little to worry about at the time. However there was to be another twist to this trivial little story. When Leah had accompanied me to my appointment to set up the vasectomy, she had visited her oncologist. She had these regular visits but they had been very similar of late and the results had been coming back very good for Leah. She had done a test on that day. The results of this test came back indicating that Leah's cancer was estrogen receptive. This meant that the chance of the cancer returning was high due to the production of estrogen in Leah's body. To rectify this it was decided the best measure would be for Leah to have a hysterectomy. All this was discovered not long after my vasectomy. So my previous procedure had, in the end, been unnecessary and Leah booked in for her operation. She was facing another major operation and I had just had my little five minute procedure but we still managed a huge laugh at this comical situation. A few days later Leah had the hysterectomy. She then came home to recover from yet another operation, more invasive surgery on a body that had already endured so much. But as per usual she took it all in her stride. One thing was for certain. This was the ultimate birth control!

Soon after these two operations life seemed to revert back to normal. A few changes had been made but we had fewer distractions on the health front now and began enjoying other facets of our lives. One episode brought us back down to earth with a thud. We had been invited to this wonderful party. It was a magnificent catered event at the stunning home of some friends of ours. To give you an idea of the type of house and the style of party I will point out some interesting facts. The couple who were having the party had bought the house several months beforehand. They wanted to turn the house into a two storey home but the neighbours objected. So instead of making the house two storey they just raised the roof of the entire house by about 1 metre to provide more light and space and to annoy the same neighbours ever so slightly. This house had a stunning kitchen area, encased by glass that led onto a gorgeous pool and courtyard. This area was where the party was held. We had a ball. We hadn't had a night out like that for ages. They offered lots of wine and food and there was plenty of dancing. We let our hair down quite a bit that night. However at about 1am Leah began to feel quite unwell. At first we thought it may have been a bit of indigestion or something similar. However it got worse. Leah said it was like really bad heart burn but it wouldn't ease up. She ended up doubled over in pain. Soon after we decided we should call an ambulance. This was to be our mode of transport from the party. Leah ended up in the emergency department at the hospital. She was admitted and numerous tests were done. It was now about 4am. We shared the ward with a number of drunken revelers who had suffered due to excessive alcohol consumption. This was not an ideal environment to end our lovely evening out. Leah was sent for some X rays and more prodding and probing. The problem turned out to be a blood clot on the lung. It could have killed her. If this clot had moved through the blood stream and into the brain it could have been devastating. Luckily we caught it in time. Leah was prescribed blood thinners to try and alleviate the clot. This was a scary night but also a frightening episode in our lives. Leah's other ailments had been a slow process during diagnosis and then the follow up treatment. Even though it was unwanted at least we could plan our lives around the solution. This clot was a different scenario. This health scare had been pretty much immediate and the consequences could have been fatal. Leah now had another thing to monitor and control with the aid of more drugs. The resultant health issues associated with cancer are quite often worse than the actual disease. The treatments used in controlling cancer can have serious implications on the body. Leah hadn't really had any issues with either of these things previously but now we had seen it, experienced it and she had lived through it. It had frightened us so much. What more did Leah have to endure? Leah now had another pill to take. One thing worked on one aspect of Leah's health but the side effects created another issue. She would almost rattle as she walked with all the medication she was on. The doctors would have to monitor her blood now as well as all the other things already being checked on a regular basis. One thing we had learned through this experience is that quite often the cancer doesn't actually kill people. What causes the damage is the associated effects on the body that crop up as a result of the cancer or the treatments that the body has to endure. This was highlighted in a book we read called "cancer - why are we still dying for a cure?" This book looked at the few options available for treatment for cancer and the dire impact these treatments may have on the patient. Patients with normally healthy organs failing due to extra pressure put on them by the cancer. It also looked at the effects of these harsh treatments on the body. It also talked of the impact most treatments had on parts of the body not even affected by cancer. The body also had to filter caustic chemicals from the patient having a huge impact on these organs. We had met a number of people who had refused treatment and just wanted to live out their final time without the invasiveness of any treatment regimes prescribed. These people wanted quality of life, with family and friends, in their final time with cancer. It got us thinking and learning. We also started enquiring and asking. We realised how ignorant we were. This was the most critical time in Leah's life and we knew nothing. We needed to know more. So a night out with some friends and a bit of dancing had created another life changing twist.

# Chapter Eight

# Moving to paradise

The other thing we had spoken about since our return from the honeymoon was the fact that we had just slotted back into our regular routine. Our friends were still the same. The house was the same. Our day to day routine was still the same. I thought this was fine. I felt safe in our little world. However, everything that Leah had been through and the things she had encountered, she wanted more. What was the purpose of life? To work until you retire and then try and enjoy it? To me these thoughts seemed silly but when faced with the prospect of not making it to retirement I guess they were perfectly natural. But how could we change this?

We had a bit of a brainstorming session. Leah's family was Dutch on her mother's side and we loved Holland so we discussed moving there to live. This would be huge. It would bring a change of culture and lifestyle. It may sound bizarre to suddenly be thinking like this but we felt we had to put it out there. I came home from work one day and

Leah asked, "How about we move to Amsterdam?" Sure, why not? I like spontaneity. If you think too clearly about things then maybe they won't happen. We tried not to let logic take over. So we started planning but it was going to be extremely difficult to arrange. At our age it was going to be so hard to get visas and work permits and the like. As Leah's family from Holland was on her mother's side she didn't qualify for a family visa as it was only based on the father's side of the family. Leah's dad was Australian so that didn't help. The international school was very expensive and the prospect of finding accommodation, furniture and moving all that way was starting to appear quite daunting. We had made so many difficult decisions over the last few years that we lost interest in this idea quite quickly due to how hard this was beginning to look. We then changed our destination to Spain. We had loved our time there. I liked the concept of living in a country where another language was spoken. I had always wanted to go to a Spanish speaking country and just live there and learn the language. We had looked at this idea years ago but cancer put an end to that. Now we found cancer was the reason for planning a similar trip. Unfortunately Spain had similar barriers to Holland.

My grandfather was born in Scotland so we investigated the prospect of me applying for the right of abode in the UK and using that for a base to travel to European destinations to work and live. However, even with the appropriate permits, this plan had the same difficulties to overcome. The Australian dollar was very weak at the time so that was another consideration as we had spent quite a bit of money in the last couple of years just with Leah's treatment, associated costs and a wedding. We came to the conclusion that this plan was not appropriate. It had been a lovely distraction. But it was pushed to one side. Leah was crushed and frustrated. But at least she was healthy. We had to focus on that. So our seemingly mundane life, which I would take any day, resumed. It was during this time that a friend came for a visit. She had just come back from living on Hamilton Island in the Whitsundays off the North Queensland coast. She had loved the experience and suggested we could look into that as a compromise. We both liked the idea. It sounded amazing. We would need no permits, visas or extra cash as it is part of Australia. We decided to investigate. We had accrued some frequent flier points from our honeymoon trip so we decided to go up to Hamilton Island for the weekend to check it out. We went on our own and left the children with their grandparents. We flew up on the Friday afternoon and as soon as we landed we knew we were moving to this dream destination. At the airport, which is actually on the island, you walk off the plane, onto the tarmac and in to the terminal. The mix of tropical heat, palm trees and the aviation fuel smell was just magical. We were hooked.

We had made arrangements to meet with the Human Resources manager, Louise, who was going to spend some time with us on the Saturday. So we checked in to the hotel and just enjoyed the evening. It felt like a second honeymoon. No children. No Pauline. We were alone in a tropical paradise. So it was exotic cocktails, palm trees, amazing sand and beach and a relaxing, romantic weekend. On the Saturday we met with Louise. She was amazing. She took us around Hamilton Island on her golf buggy which is the mode of transport for everyone. We went up to the lookout and saw the stunning views in all directions. This was like a dream. We went to most of the food and beverage outlets, the school, the kindy and the quaint little church. She showed us the staff accommodation on the island and then she took us to a restaurant and bought us lunch. We sat overlooking the ocean on one side and the resort pool on the other. Louise was an amazing woman. She did explain, though, that the process to living on the island was to first get a job and then the accommodation was provided. Louise also mentioned that Hamilton Island was being sold so there weren't the positions vacant at present so the process of moving would be virtually impossible. We disagreed. We had dealt with impossible before. She laughed but we were adamant that we were moving to Hamilton Island and would make it happen. We finished our lovely meal and then thanked Louise for all her help and generosity and then we continued with our romantic weekend. We went swimming, we snoozed, had a few naughty cocktails and took beautiful long walks. This was quality alone time without a care in the world. We hadn't had that for quite some time. But quite quickly the weekend was over. We headed back to the airport. We savoured the final tropical sights, sounds and smells and said farewell for the time being. We would return very soon. But in the meantime we headed back to Melbourne, picked up the children from their grandparents and told everyone we were moving to a tropical paradise.

Before investigating Hamilton Island or even having Hamilton Island as a thought we had already been planning our next adventure. This had been a dream for some time. Leah was good at planning these things and then setting a budget so we could achieve our goal. Leah wanted to experience a white Christmas as a family. I know this is beginning to sound a lot like a bucket list but it was actually just a need for Leah to experience as much as possible while also taking her mind off her illness, which had behaved for quite some time now. We had already arranged the trip to Canada for our white Christmas which would be in December and January. This was another thing we agreed to do with the saving of not having to move to Europe. So we would do this trip to Canada and then move to Hamilton Island in late January. What an exciting period of our lives this was. This was exactly what Leah needed. Many wishes were coming true for her. But she definitely deserved it. She had endured so much with this rotten disease and missed out on so much as well. She had been denied important family time. She had missed time for herself as a woman. She quite often missed out on activities with the children and we, as a couple, had missed out on so much. Leah was determined not to just sit at home and contemplate her health and her future. She was going to determine her future. She didn't want to wait and see what the future was to be. She wanted to create it. It was tough for her and I had to support her all the way through. We were both working most of the time. We were great at budgeting. We didn't indulge in vices that cost too much, except for travel. So we were able to make these dreams come true. We were creating life long memories. These were unique experiences. We were enjoying life with the children in magical settings to lessen the impact that cancer had created in our lives. We were evening up the score if you like. We were about to cram a lifetime of memories into a very short time. I had never been so nervous in my life. A lot of this was way out of our comfort zone. But then again cancer was not in many people's comfort zone either. It may have been out of our comfort zone but what a great feeling this was. This was so much better than dealing with the unknown in a reactive manner as you do so often when cancer is in your lives.

Soon it was time for our trip to Canada. We flew to Vancouver first. What a great city. It was winter so it would get dark mid afternoon. We walked through snow. It was slippery. The streets had fairy lights and we dressed for the weather. You could walk past churches and hear caroling. The hotels had Christmas themes and it felt just right for Christmas. The Hyatt hotel in the city had a huge gingerbread man that was 20 feet tall and was surrounded by a gingerbread village that local school children had created. We sat in the hotel's coffee shop and drank hot chocolate and admired our surroundings. We spent time walking in the snow, rugged up in really warm winter clothing. Ski jackets, muffs, hiking boots, long Johns. We had come prepared. It was quite often 20 below zero. We visited little markets and the local zoo with white Beluga whales. It was a winter wonderland. We took a quaint little ferry over to Granville Island where the artists create and sell their wares. We loved Vancouver. We loved the

Canadian breakfast at the hotel. We indulged in waffles, bacon, maple syrup and other yummy treats that set us up for a day in the cold. We then flew to Calgary and got ready for hitting the snow. We spent a few days there and it was a bit colder than Vancouver. We bought a little toboggan and practiced on some gentle slopes. It still wasn't Christmas. But it was just around the corner. We caught a bus to Banff. This is where we would spend Christmas. Banff is a truly magical town. This was the perfect town for a white Christmas. It had snowed quite heavily in November but hadn't snowed much since. There was a covering of icy and slightly dirty snow but Rebecca wished it would snow again for Christmas. We hoped for the same. Banff was gorgeous. It was a little village that would be perfect for our white Christmas. We visited the Chateau Fairmont hotel which was like a medieval castle but was, in fact, a glorious exclusive resort. We could go through to the back of the hotel where they had frozen lakes and we ice skated and played ice hockey with the locals and tobogganed down the slopes. We laughed and screamed and had so much fun. This was a winter wonderland. Upon conclusion we would adjourn to the lobby where complimentary warm apple cider was on offer with a cinnamon stick and we would warm up while we waited for a taxi to drop us back at our hotel. We went to a few local church services and the locals were so welcoming and would invite us to enjoy tea and a biscuit with them and we would exchange stories. It felt like how Christmas really should be. The children were so excited on Christmas eve but also so tired that they fell to sleep early. When we woke Christmas morning it was snowing. Rebecca's wish had come true. This freshened up the village and it looked perfect. The village was pure white. Moose and reindeer were wandering down the main street.  We went down stairs to the restaurant to have breakfast. We went through the lobby and past the Christmas tree which had presents underneath. The children were still in their pajamas and scurried off to see if any of the presents had their names on them. Of course they did. They tore open the presents and the joy on their faces was priceless. They had been through a lot in the last few years and this erased some of the bad experiences for the moment. Leah's present, from me for Christmas, was an airline ticket which was for all of us to fly to Toronto and then visit Niagara Falls. It hadn't been part of our plans due to the cost of organising this from Australia. But once in Canada I could get some great deals and it was able to be done and it made a great surprise for Christmas. We had a lovely Christmas breakfast, spent the day playing with new toys, wandered the streets of Banff and finished with a lovely Christmas dinner back at the hotel restaurant. It had been a Christmas to remember. How could we ever top it? Christmas in Banff was the best ever. On Boxing Day we then moved on to Jasper for a few days. It was the coldest place on our trip and a bit more rustic than the other places but very nice as well. We went to the movies in an historic old cinema and we did more ice skating on the frozen lake. Next stop was Lake Louise. We were to have New Years Eve at the Chateau Fairmont at Lake Louise which is an amazing resort right on the lake. The lake was frozen at this time of the year, but offered lovely views of frozen waterfalls and glaciers and was, again, quite magical. The chefs had made an ice castle on the frozen lake which lit up at night. We were able to go on horse drawn sleigh rides over the frozen lake. This place was like something out of a fairytale and was such a memorable experience. Christmas had been amazing and this was such a unique experience as well. To see Leah's reaction to all this made me so proud and happy. We had wanted this to be a once in a lifetime experience and it was living up to that expectation. The adventures we were having and the joy experienced by the children was unforgettable. Canada was magical. Melbourne and the horrible disease called cancer seemed so far away. After an extremely special New Years Eve we travelled back to Calgary for the flight to Toronto. We stayed there for a week and went on a trip to Niagara Falls which also felt like a dream come true, another once in a lifetime experience. We actually felt quite insignificant next to the majestic Niagara Falls and the experience really helped us contemplate what we had been through as a family. It also enabled us to be thankful for all the wonderful times we had been lucky enough to have in our relatively short time together. After Toronto and the wonderful Niagara Falls we flew to Vancouver again and then on to Whistler. One of the owners of the hotel where Leah and I had worked and met owned a property at Whistler. So we were able to catch up with him and his family and we got to stay in the amazing resort town of Whistler. Whistler was also a winter wonderland. But it was also quite different to the other places we had been to. Rebecca did some ski lessons and had a day skiing and we all did a skidoo trip over the crest of the mountains. We had a lovely dinner at our friend's house. We loved Canada. We didn't want to leave. Canada had given us everlasting and wonderful memories. This stage of our lives was a time when Leah was well, happy and full of life. It was a time when we were a lucky, happy family without a worry in the world.

While we were away in Canada, Louise from Hamilton Island contacted us. There were no jobs available still but she had a solution. One of the privately owned units had become available for rent and she offered it to us. We didn't need to have a job to rent privately and as we were going to rent out our house in Melbourne, we jumped at the offer. The rent from our house would pay for the rent of the Hamilton Island unit. This was perfect. So we left Canada happy in the knowledge that our plan to live in paradise had come to fruition. We were leaving minus 30 degree temperatures and heading for a humid and tropical 30 degree climate. Our wonderful Canadian experience had come to an end and we were heading back to Australia for a new life.

We got back to Australia and had a few things to take care of. Leah had a few appointments before our move. Her oncologist had suggested a drug called Herceptin. This was a cancer inhibitor. The cancer cells could return but Herceptin would prevent the cells from joining together and forming clusters or tumours. It appeared not to have any side effects and could be administered from either Proserpine or Mackay hospitals which were relatively close to where we were moving.  It was good to finally get a treatment that had no side effects. We were so relaxed. We were happy and we were leaving the mess of cancer behind. We were moving to a beautiful spot that would be beneficial to all of us. The children would be able to escape the environment of their mum having such severe highs and lows. Leah could really concentrate on her health by including such activities as yoga, meditation and diet in the tropical paradise which would be life on Hamilton Island. I would worry about how it would all work when we got there. We were sure that work would follow. We moved up to Hamilton Island and the unit we were moving into was a few days off being ready so we stayed at the Whitsunday apartments for a few days. These are resort style but had cooking facilities and larger living areas which suited our needs. We spent a few days just enjoying resort life. We swam with the kids in the many resort pools. We spent time on the beach. We took in the sights of this tropical island resort. This was now our home. We got the children organised with school and kindy. Bec was going to Hamilton Island State School which was just down the road from where we would be living. It was a school of 50 students. Bim would attend the kindy which was really a childcare centre like a kindergarten back home. The kindy was just down the road as well. There were swimming pools everywhere. The beach was just across the road and everyone got around in golf buggies. We were set. It didn't take long to settle in to this lifestyle. It was all perfect. The kids thought they were on a never ending holiday. But they soon got a big shock. They had to go back to school. The first day of school included a new uniform for the children. It was green. They travelled to school in a golf buggy. This was already so new and exciting for them. Leah was so well during this time and actually beaming with the excitement of our new life. She was healthy and happy and got to see the children attend their first day at a new school and kindy. It truly was a special time. But we had to head into reality as well. It was time to start to look for work. We still hadn't moved in to our new home yet. We were still living in a resort apartment. The next few days were spent arranging the move into our new unit and trying to find work. The children settled in well. They had already made numerous friends. However school life was a bit difficult to ease into. The resort lifestyle could be quite transient. Because of this many of the settled kids were a bit apprehensive about taking in new friends. They were a bit concerned that new friends may leave if their parents decided to move off the island. We assured them all that this would not be the case for us and things progressed quite well. Our unit was in a complex that had numerous families which was great. It turned out to be a very supportive environment. It was interesting that living in a resort we were still able to have such a neighbourhood feeling. We were happy. The children were happy. This had been a great move.

We went over to the mainland on the ferry to check out the towns over there and meet with doctors, oncologists and to check out facilities. The trip on the ferry took nearly an hour. However it was such a wonderful trip. We'd stop at the other resort islands to drop off or pick up passengers. The ferry even had to stop to allow migrating whales to pass at certain times of the year. Airlie Beach was the first town we got to which was just a tourist Mecca. It accommodated mainly back packers but had some nice things to visit such as a lovely lagoon and the local markets. Airlie Beach had a few resorts as well as local residents so it was a nice place to visit. Cannonvale was just next to it. This was more residential and had the shopping centre and more schools and facilities. Proserpine was about an hour away and had another airport, bigger shopping area and of course the hospital.

Mackay which was about another hour away was a big centre with a bigger hospital and more infrastructure but would only be needed on an occasional basis. Leah would have to travel to the mainland periodically to get to her appointments to undertake her usual regular checks. Leah still needed many appointments, blood tests, scans and meetings with doctors and her new oncologist. Even though cancer hadn't been spoken of for some time she still needed monitoring to ensure it didn't come back. So moving to the Whitsundays had been done after quite a bit of research. We had researched everything in and around the area. Even though we were a long way from things, there was nothing we could not get. Things that weren't readily available we could get sent by the post. I could even get our regular brand of coffee posted up. Our new life had begun and we were quite organised already. While the kids got settled at school we took a few weeks to just be together as a couple and relax. We would swim, meet new friends, have the odd lunch, chill out and generally just enjoy what the island offered. This was quite a positive time for us. But soon it was back to reality. I really just wanted to work at the Beachouse restaurant. I would have liked the change. The Beachouse had the main resort pool on one side and the ocean on the other. I would be happy mixing drinks and really enjoying work as part of our new lifestyle. I met the food and beverage manager and submitted my resume. As I mentioned earlier the resort had quite a transient workforce so they were licking their lips at the prospect of a long term employee. The food and beverage manager took my resume to the Human Resources department for approval and he told me to expect to have employment by the afternoon. I was so happy. Leah also had an interview with the Beach club. This was the resorts 5 star accommodation at the time. Guests had their own personal staff to pick them up, ferry them around, make reservations, bring meals and other requests. It had its own pool that others could not access and its own private part of the beach with "special" lounges and towels and facilities. Leah got the job and started straight away. She loved it. I had a hiccup with my situation. After my resume was presented to the Human Resources department it was noted that my training background featured prominently. They no longer wanted me for the restaurant position but to head up the new training department. This job would be Monday to Friday and in an air conditioned office. Leah and I chatted about this and thought it would be good for the children as it didn't involve shift work and would make arranging school a lot easier. Done.

So we both started new careers and new lives and it was all very exciting. I would finish work at 5pm and by 5 past we could be at the beach, as a family, living life. This really was paradise. Leaving a secure job, great friends, close family and the comforts of our previous situation took a vast amount of courage. It had been scary. But it had also been one of the most liberating things I had ever done. It was a big move especially as Leah was settled into her cancer routine in Melbourne. However the unknown was exciting. We had a new spark in our lives. We were now in control of cancer and had refused to stay tied to the constraints cancer forces into many peoples' lives. We felt free. Every day was a new adventure. We were Ash and Leah and the kids, not poor Leah, who had cancer and her family. We had names and faces again. Bec and Bim loved the island life. We had a few teething problems but once established we could never go back. Leah and I immediately took up outrigger canoeing. This is a big pastime on Hamilton Island and they hold a big regatta each year. This would keep us fit and enable us to meet new friends. As we lived in a tropical paradise we had lots of visitors and we also did lots of exploring by ourselves. When friends came up we went and had breakfast with the koalas. The kids loved it. This was very special. We made amazing lifelong new friends. We ate out, we entertained at home, we snorkeled, went boating, travelled up to places like Townsville, Bowen, Cairns and Port Douglas. All these places were in Far North Queensland so we decided to do as much as possible while we were up that way. We went out to the

Great Barrier Reef and Whitehaven beach. These are iconic destinations within the Whitsundays. We were blessed.

# Chapter Nine

# Leah's first helicopter ride

My cousin, who lived just out of Cairns in far North Queensland, had a wedding to attend on the mainland just over from Hamilton Island. She decided to pop over for the day and visit. I hadn't seen Elsie in years and had never met her husband. Obviously it was the first time also for Leah. They caught the ferry over and we met them and showed them around. The kids went to the pool and we went and sat by the side of the pool and caught up. It was beautiful weather and such a nice day for all of us. We then went back to our unit for lunch. It was great to catch up and for strangers to meet for the first time. It was a fun day. While I was getting the lunch ready Leah felt a bit funny and needed to go for a lie down. She had been fine all of the time since moving to paradise. Leah had been enjoying work, participating at the school, being part of the kindy and our social life. Maybe she was just a little bit tired on this day. She excused herself and went for a lie down. I continued making lunch but thought I'd check on her. As I entered the room she started convulsing. This was shocking. In all the episodes we had encountered previously I had never been confronted by anything such as this. I tried to comfort her. I really didn't know what to do. I had never felt so helpless. We had a medical centre and security department on the island so I rang them. I tried to comfort Leah while we waited. Chris came straight away. He calmed her down and gave her something to calm the shaking. He had come over in the resort ambulance so he loaded Leah into that. She had stabilised quite a bit but was still reacting in an abnormal way. They transported Leah by ambulance to the airport where a helicopter awaited. She was to be flown over to Mackay hospital. This was scary. I went back to the unit. Tim and Elsie were still there. They were concerned and stayed to make sure everything was alright. Then, once it had been established everything was under some sort of control, they went down to the ferry for the trip back to the mainland. It was not the best way to spend the day on a tropical island. But they were caring and concerned and after it had been established that Leah was alright they thought it best to depart. I felt quite alone at this stage. Leah quite often went to the mainland but was always back by the last ferry, around 6 pm. I thought that this time she would be away for some time. I tried to keep busy while I waited to find out what had happened. I had a few domestic chores to take care of so I did these, as Leah went in the helicopter, to take my mind off things. However in about 15 minutes the phone rang and it was the hospital letting me know Leah had arrived safely, was feeling better and was comfortable and being looked after. We were living on an island and the trip to hospital was quicker than if we were living in the suburbs of Melbourne and an ambulance was required. I was relieved. I explained all of what had happened so far to the children. They were obviously a bit scared but confident their mum would be fine. Over the next few days Leah had to undergo numerous tests and scans. The result of all of these scans was a huge and unexpected shock and a great setback. She had brain tumours. Lots of them.

Leah rang and we discussed the options. Well she only had one option really. The only thing they could offer was to schedule whole head radiation. This would take about a month. It was decided she would be best going to Melbourne and staying with her parents and getting the radiation at a hospital close by. We set it all up and Leah flew out of Mackay to Melbourne. The children didn't get a chance to say goodbye in person as Leah had left straight from the hospital. Her parents met her, took her home and began the month long regime of looking after their daughter and ensuring she made it to all of her treatment sessions. They would stay and wait and then take her home, feed her, look after her and comfort her. Knowing Leah was being well cared for  was a blessing and a weight off my mind. Nothing like being looked after by mum to make things all better. I still had to work and look after the children. I don't think I could have done it anywhere else but Hamilton Island. Nothing was more than 2 minutes away. In the mornings I would get the children off to school, make their lunches and then I'd go to work. I would head home on my afternoon tea break to ensure they got home from school and kindy, get them a snack and drink, set up homework for Bec and then head back to work. Just after 5pm I would be home and then get dinner ready and that's how our life went for the month. Our neighbours were great. As I mentioned it was a very supportive, family orientated area of the island in which we lived. This made things a lot less of a worry for me. We would ring Leah at night or she'd ring us. We missed her. She missed us. She had been away for  a short time before, when she went to the Gawler Foundation, but she was in good health at that time. This time she had left in an emergency situation and was then away for a month. It was different, it felt different. It was not right. This was the first time she had been away from us for so long. It was a difficult time. We faced the unexpected again. I felt for our poor kids. They were being subjected to the unknown again. It was tough on Leah going through all this but it was almost as tough for Bec and Blm to be without their mum for so long again. However as we were so busy with work and school the month went fairly quickly. Before we knew it Leah was coming home. The kids were so excited. They made her welcome back gifts and cards. We took the buggy to the airport to meet Leah. At the airport you can almost wait on the tarmac. It's pretty casual and quite small and usually only one plane lands at a time. The plane arrived and we waited for the passengers to disembark. We waited in the area where the passengers file past to go to the baggage claim area. We waited and we waited. No Leah. Or so we thought. Had she missed the plane? Had something gone wrong that we weren't aware of? No, nothing had happened. She had actually walked past us and we hadn't realised. She was behind us, waiting for some help and she turned and yelled to us. We hadn't noticed her. We turned and saw a frail old lady who resembled someone of 80 years of age, not our Leah. She shuffled rather than walked. It was distressing but we ran over and gave her a hug to welcome her home. It was difficult for the children to see their mum like this. The radiation had really taken its toll. She was a shell of the woman who had left in a helicopter over a month ago. What had they done to her? This treatment had been the worst as far as side effects had been on Leah. It was horrendous. But if it worked it would all be worth it, right?


We were in paradise but Leah was in a haze. She could hardly function and required a cocktail of drugs to reduce the effects of the radiation. Obviously she could not work so the financial stress began again. We applied for a carers benefit but that was rejected as Leah was not unwell enough to allow me to qualify for this. She was also not eligible for the disability pension. So I continued to work but now I would duck home at morning tea time, lunch time and afternoon tea time to ensure Leah was alright, get her a juice or something to eat and help her try to get better and stronger. The children were great with helping out around home. Hamilton Island was actually a great spot for Leah to recover. The warmth was great for her. The beach was not far and she quite often just sat in the sun. She would spend time under a palm tree, meditating, sleeping and resting up. Our friends were amazing. Some would drop by and give Leah a ride if she needed to get somewhere. Our neighbours on one side were a group of young girls and a more generous group they could not be. They would bake for us. They would come and babysit. The girls would help clean and pop in to see if we needed assistance. Leah needed regular trips to the hospital to check on her progress. Obviously I needed to go over with her. I spoke with Leah's oncologists and asked how this had happened. Where did these tumours come from? Apparently the Herceptin which Leah was on was not perfect. One of the issues was its molecular structure. It was a cancer inhibitor but was molecularly sized so that it could not penetrate the brains protective barrier and therefore could only protect the body and not the brain. The cancer cells have a pre disposition to form tumours and the only place they could do this was the brain. Great! It seemed a bit harder to treat the tumours in the brain and with many more side effects. A new battle had begun. It took quite a few months for Leah to get much better. Her muscle tone had wasted quite a bit. She was weaker. But as we ate well and nurtured her body and spirit we saw a gradual improvement in all aspects of her wellbeing.  What did the future hold for us now? This was one of the most difficult times for Leah, myself and the children. It was new and uncertain. We had gained the upper hand but now that had been taken away from us. The great memories of the last year or so were beginning to feel like a distant memory. We had advanced so much yet now we were further behind than ever. We needed to do something. But what?

# Chapter Ten

# The ashram and SpongeBob Squarepants

This was all a new twist in an already unpalatable situation. After several months Leah was feeling a lot better. Now it was time to help restore the health and vitality to the neglected areas of her body due to the severity of the impact of the radiation treatment. She also had to go for follow up scans to ascertain how effective the radiation had been. I took a day off work and we drove to Mackay for the day so Leah could have the scans on her brain. The wait for the results was agonising. This was scarier than any of the previous times. The news was shattering. There was no change in her condition. She still had 9 tumours. The radiation on the brain hadn't done anything. Except reduce Leah to a shell of her former self. This was extremely upsetting. Worse was to follow. We learned that radiation on the brain can only be done once as there is a risk of brain damage. What are we subjecting cancer patients to?

So now any further radiation was off the list as an option. Thank God for that, in a funny way. I thought the treatment was almost worse than the disease. But now we needed to know what Leah's options were. The response was mind numbing. They told us that there was nothing they could offer. What did that mean? Weren't we in the 21st century? Here was a vital young mum in the prime of her life and the doctors had no options to offer? I thought it was a joke. We donate millions every year to cancer charities and our treatment options had just run out! I wasn't going to accept that. I rang the doctors and oncologists in Melbourne and even Sydney. There was nothing. We did hear of one doctor in Melbourne who someone suggested could help. We rang and he asked for Leah's scans. They had a device called the Linear Accelerator. I hadn't heard of this before. Drugs were all we were offered previously. We enquired about the Linear Accelerator but it wasn't versatile enough for Leah's situation. It can only really treat 3 tumours, size was also an issue and they liked to follow up with whole head radiation and as she had already had this once they don't do it again. Again, they mentioned brain damage. This was the second time we had been advised of this. What sort of treatments are we subjecting people to? Surely there are better options around? However as we asked we discovered that the options had run out. Leah had been given a death sentence. We were perplexed, empty and shattered. This couldn't be happening. Lots of people get cancer and survive. Leah was going to be one of them right? But how could we get her better? Could we look at alternative medicine? Maybe a miracle? Any option would do. But she was given nothing. It was time to look outside the square. We didn't know where though at present. We had to go home to ponder this latest development. The drive home was very solemn. We were in a daze. It seemed like the drive took so many hours. The time just dragged. We just wanted to wake up from this bad dream.

We had made a few contacts through Leah's previous experiences. It was now time to utilise some of these. One chap had been through a great experience of going to India and visiting a guru over there. We researched this and discovered that for a number of decades people such as Goldie Hawn and Richard Gere and millions of others had visited this spiritual man named Sai Baba. Leah was the spiritual one and as we had no options from conventional means we decided that any possibility from a different area couldn't hurt. We put the wheels in motion. Leah's parents came up to Hamilton Island to mind the children and we booked the trip to Bangalore in India for a two week residency at the ashram in which Sai Baba resides. Our friend Cath, who ran a hotel in Victoria and was a bit stressed at the time, decided to join us. The company and support would do us the world of good. Cath was coming from Melbourne so we would meet her in India. We had to fly down to Sydney and catch a flight from there to Singapore then a connecting flight to Bangalore in India. While we were going from the domestic to international terminal in Sydney we passed a stand offering free postcards advertising various products. One of these cards was a bright yellow SpongeBob Squarepants card. We decided to grab the whole pile. We had also been given lots of money to take to some orphanages in India to offer some help to the young children there. Friends and family had organised this so that we could use the time over in India to help others as well. Good Karma. While we waited at the international terminal for our flight we wrote a SpongeBob Squarepants postcard to Bec and Bim and posted them from Sydney so they would get them in time and let them know how much we already missed them and that we loved them. I don't know how Leah coped with her month away from the children when she had been getting her radiation. It was difficult for me already after just several hours. These are the effects of cancer that aren't really noticed from the outside. Small sacrifices but as the time goes by the small sacrifices add up to huge losses. Our kids had already missed so much. But they had also experienced so much due to the illness. Bim had never seen Leah with long flowing curly blonde hair which is what she had when we first met. Bec had lost important days when Leah was away or sick and wasn't able to participate in crucial times for a young girl. We had to make all this right. Could India help us?

We arrived in Bangalore, in the southern part of India, early in the morning. We were amazed at what confronted us initially. We stepped out of the airport and were met by beggars, lepers, hustle and bustle. It was mad, hot and chaotic. We found a driver and he drove us off to the ashram. The roads were crazy, traffic was maniacal and there appeared to be no road rules. It took a while to get to the ashram. Luckily the car was air conditioned. We checked in upon arrival and retired to our rooms. They were very basic. There was no carpet, just plain concrete walls and a very basic bathroom. But we did discover that the material things in life weren't important here. Sai Baba led worship sessions six times a day starting at about 4 am. I never made it to any of the really early ones but Leah did. We would go together for the next one at about 8am. The ashram had thousands of people flocking from all over the world. Many locals attended also. Food was served in a big dining hall in which we all had to participate at some stage in preparation and clean up. There were a number of these dining halls around the facility which we could choose from. All the food was vegetarian and, of course, no alcohol. Male and female residents did not fraternise during meals and we were ushered into separate dining areas for male and female. Cath and Leah would go in one direction and I would head in the other direction. We sat on large communal tables, thanked the Gods for the meal and then ate. Silence was practiced at this time. But before and afterwards we would have a chat. Many didn't speak English but we still communicated. The meals were brilliant. There was lots of chickpea dishes, dahl, rice, great breads, lassi's, yummy milky coffee and the like. After eating we would meet up outside in the beautiful surroundings again. There was a lot to see. The gardens were magical and featured unusual and stunning plants. The ponds had exotic water lilies and other aquatic plants. The ashram had fairly basic facilities. Again it was to cater for the bare necessities. There was a post office. It also had a supermarket that was only open for an hour at a time and again males and females couldn't shop together. Outside of the ashram was a village. It contained little cafes, stores, vendors and more hustle and bustle. It was very colourful and exciting. Ladies would thread cotton through amazingly bright flower heads to form necklaces that we could buy. We would venture over each day to one of the cafes and have a Fanta or Sprite. It would only cost about 20 cents and then we'd get a refund on the bottle. The attire in the ashram and beyond was the punjabi. Soft free flowing cloth outfits and a pair of slippers or sandals. As Leah had lost her hair during her radiation treatment she looked quite at home in this environment. She even painted a tiny red dot on her forehead. The spiritual services were massive. We would queue up for about an hour. Thousands attended each session. Males and females were segregated again. You went through metal detectors before entering the temple to ensure no weapons were taken in. They are extremely passionate about their spiritual idols in this country. Anyone jealous or with differing spiritual beliefs may be tempted to do some harm to someone such as Sai Baba if they didn't believe in his ways. So security was essential. After passing through the security check we would sit on the stone floor. We learnt early on to purchase a stadium cushion from one of the shops in the village. Without a cushion all the sitting would render ones backside quite numb. The chatter prior to Sai Baba entering was intense. Thousands of people, who were there six times a day, were catching up like they hadn't seen each other for four years not just four hours. It took a while for all the participants to be ushered through security and into the temple so the waiting was the hardest part. I would usually be way up the back. Leah would get right up front as we discovered, that due to having an illness, she got preferential seating. So the chatter would be almost deafening and then Sai Baba would approach in his golf cart from his residence. He would climb the stairs to the platform and, as soon as he was visible, the chatter would stop in an instant. It was an amazing experience. He would then look around the area and as his gaze came into the general vicinity of the worshippers, they would reach up with their hands and grab his strength, gaze or power in the palm of their hands. This was another amazing experience. His sermon, speech, oration, whatever you would like to call it, was all in Indian. So I didn't understand much. I didn't need to. The power he projected and the manner in which he delivered it was awe inspiring to the participants. He didn't do much for me or Leah though. It may have been the language barrier. It could have been that we were novices. I am not sure. I thought there would have been more of an aura or a presence. There obviously was but I didn't experience it from the great man himself. The atmosphere provided some amazing sensations. The environment we were in was quite special. I got more from watching the others around me. Maybe two weeks wasn't long enough. Most of these people had experienced this event for years and throughout many generations. I was more amazed at the impact he had on these people. They were mostly people, who had very little materialistically, but were immensely happy. They were all much richer than I.

Leah got to meet Sai Baba. He was a man in his 80's who had a huge following and had done so much for the community. Some people got to go on stage and touch him and this was where the miracles happened apparently. A miracle didn't happen for Leah but it was an amazing experience all the same. The local people had very little. Most of the locals were very poor. But I could tell they were so rich in other aspects of their lives. The rich Westerners, like us, were looking for other benefits of attending the ashram. I think many envied the local Indian population and the impact this experience had on them. Many of the Westerners were wealthy but were obviously searching for something money can't buy. An example of the social aspect of all this on the locals was witnessed near our room at the ashram. Next to our accommodation was, what we called, the chook house. We had a private room whereas the chook house had mats on the dirt floor and slept about one hundred people. When we first got to our room we could here this noise reminiscent of kookaburras, or a chicken battery farm. But it was all the locals in this shared accommodation, who had no TV or distractions, so it was just a place for catching up, chatting, laughing and on mass it was powerful. We had a lights out time and when that came upon us the noise from the chook house would cease in an instant. It was truly amazing stuff.

We enjoyed our time at the ashram even if it had not delivered the miracle we had hoped for. It was time to go. Sai Baba had not been the saviour we had hoped for. In fact I think he was a bit old. I could imagine the charisma he may have had back in the 1970's and 80's but he did little to inspire us. He appeared to be a lovely man. In fact, while I have been writing this, he actually passed away and I felt a strong loss. I saw that the Dalai Lama wrote a lovely message of praise about Sai Baba. One thing we couldn't deny was the effect he had on thousands of people every day. The money we paid for the experience goes to the local town and the schools, services and hospital were well funded due to Sai Baba. I learnt a lot about things I had never even pondered in life before. I read a lot about India, the religions, the people and the wonderful places in this country. The Indian people believe in reincarnation which was something we hadn't thought about prior to our visit. It gave us some comfort thinking about this aspect of life or death. Even though we didn't appear to get much physically from the experience in India we certainly grew as people and left with a lot of respect for the people and we encountered much self discovery. Leah was faced with the worst future one could possibly have. Yet we felt that this experience had helped in our progression and transition as we went forward in life. Life was simple here, the people uncomplicated and they had educated us and had such a huge impact on our lives. We would bring the children here one day so they could experience the diversity for themselves. I wanted to know more and a great introduction for me was to read a book called Holy Cow by Australian author Sarah Macdonald. She had lived in India with her ABC correspondent husband. While he was out reporting she would explore and then she put all these experiences into a wonderful book. It's funny, sad and extremely uplifting. I read it very quickly.

I know it sounds weird moving on to a cartoon character just after the uplifting experience we had just been a part of. However we left the ashram and ventured back to Bangalore for a bit of a rest and to be tourists for a few days before we went home. We booked into a cheap hotel which was actually quite nice. It had a roof top Tandoori restaurant which was a change from the segregated dining of the ashram. We shopped in the hustle bustle that was Bangalore and the surrounds. We drank gin and tonics in the afternoons. But we had business to attend to. We had collected money prior to leaving Australia which we promised we would use to help the local orphans. We were warned to not just donate the cash as it would be frittered away, misappropriated, stolen or all three. So we decided to buy things and treats that the children could use or that they needed. We got a driver who knew of a couple of orphanages we could visit and help and he drove us to them. One was set up initially in the name of Mother Theresa. The other was a more business minded orphanage. We called the residents of the latter, the lucky orphans. The children were nominated for adoption to overseas families, mainly European. They still did it pretty tough as far as facilities and standards were concerned but the futures of these kids seemed quite rosy. We got them some colouring books, plates and cups as they shared meals off one plate between three or four children at the time. We also got things like toothpaste and soap. The children ran and played and enjoyed our presence. It was gratifying to see their responses to us. The interaction with them was what was missing in their lives. They enjoyed the fact that we gave them some attention rather than the day to day interactions with the few staff they had to look after them. We were feeling good. This was all part of the experience we were after from this trip. Then we went off to the other orphanage. This was for kids who were disadvantaged and had little hope of having normal lives. Some had birth defects, others had mental issues. It was very hard to cope with. This experience was very emotional. But the children just wanted hugs and attention. There was hardly any staff and the kids lived in such crude surroundings. One little girl played in the concrete yard with a polystyrene bean bag filling ball which was being blown around by the breeze. They ate off a shared plate again and some of the less able were actually drooling in to the food others were eating. It was a devastating time for us. The orphanage was run by nuns and when we returned with a big box of utensils and treats and toys they were very grateful. I could only stay for about five minutes due to the effect the experience had on me. This was extremely overwhelming. Leah managed to stay a few minutes longer but not by much. I had never experienced anything like this. We had visited orphanages in Thailand previously where some of the children were orphans from losing parents to Aids but even that experience was easier to cope with than the despair we felt here. Leah was not happy with her lot at the moment but at least she had freedom, love and happiness in her life. These kids were very hard done by and we failed to see the justice or reason in life for them. We left with mixed emotions. When we returned home to Australia one of the first things we did was sponsor three children from overseas. Not much, I know, but an action we had to take. As we had driven through the numerous suburbs and towns to get to the orphanages, children would come up to the car and ask for money and gifts. We had the SpongeBob postcards from Sydney airport so we handed them out as we went. Most of these children wouldn't have had television but the bright yellow image of SpongeBob Squarepants was exciting for these kids who had very little. The orphans also liked them. On our return trip to the hotel, as we went through some of the areas we had passed earlier, we noted the SpongeBob cards attached to trees, posts and buildings. We had a little chuckle. It was a shallow happiness compared to the eye opening experience of visiting the orphanages. This trip had been a life changing experience. Even though it was difficult to find much joy in what we had just experienced we hoped that our participation in the children's lives and the generosity of our friends had helped brighten their day. This visit made us appreciate our children and what we had. It confirmed how much love we had for our kids. So we spent the last few days doing more touristy things such as shopping for gifts for our children and people back home. We did some sightseeing and had a few lovely meals as we enjoyed each other's company as tourists before our return home to Australia. India had truly been an amazing experience.

# Chapter 11

# Amazing discoveries and amazing new friends

We returned home to Hamilton Island hopeful that Leah had been granted a miracle by Sai Baba and the cancer had disappeared. It was great to be back home with the children and Leah's parents were so glad to see us. It was the first time I had been away from the kids for such a long time. Of course Leah was quite used to being away by now. This did not make it any easier for either of us. We had brought back gifts for our children. Indian costumes, musical instruments and trinkets from our trip. Seeing the children in the orphanages had made us miss our two so much. It made us appreciate how lucky we were. We were now able to allow life to go back to normal. This was at least our version of normal. It was our normal life on our island paradise. Leah was still off work as she was trying to regain her strength and most of her time was spent meditating, exercising and getting back to her old self. She also had her usual requirements of appointments with oncologists, doctors and specialists. I wondered what they thought of us trekking all the way over to India for a miracle. Leah was then scheduled for another scan to see where she was at. Had there been any improvement with the tumours in her brain? It was a nervous wait for the results. We were still hoping for that miracle. However the news was not good. There was still no change. The radiation that had almost killed Leah had made no difference to the tumours. Our Indian guru had provided no miracle. Leah's oncologist recommended that she return home to get her affairs in order. What does that even mean? This was devastating news and something we had not even contemplated before. Leah had written her own eulogy at The Gawler retreat but more as a sign of strength against the cancer rather than an indication of what might lie ahead. This was a very difficult time for us. We couldn't explain it all to the children but they saw our emotions fluctuate and knew something was different. They had been through so much in such short lives so far. We rang everyone we knew for assistance. We read everything we could to try and find a way to fix this seemingly unfixable situation. We looked at Blue Scorpion venom from Cuba. People in the USA go to Mexico and get Blue Scorpion venom administered as a cancer treatment. It's had some amazing results. We were impressed. After all nothing was on offer here. We rang to find some more information about it. Little farms in Cuba breed these scorpions and then they milk them for the venom. It's natural and has no side effects. It sounded better. We then rang Australian Customs to see if we could import some. The man from Customs told us that several hundred people from Australia had imported the venom and used it in their cancer treatment. It was amazing what lengths people go to for a solution. There was quite a lot of evidence, albeit not sufficient to be conclusive, of people successfully using Blue Scorpion venom to eradicate cancer. However we didn't know enough for this to be the answer just yet.

We ordered some apricot kernels. They had vitamin B17 which was good for cancer prevention. We would grind up the kernels and fill empty capsule cases and Leah would take them just like a tablet. You can get vitamin B17 administered intravenously overseas but it's not allowed in Australia. We had known of many managing their cancer with vitamin B17 so thought it may be worth a try as the doctors in Australia couldn't help anymore. The capsules of B17 became part of Leah's daily ritual. This was a ritual we were used to and felt it was making a difference. Our latest news cast some doubt on where we could go now. We were worn out. I was stressed which is very unusual for me. Leah was shattered. We needed a break.

Christmas was coming upon us and we decided to head to the Gold Coast for a break. We were spoilt. We leave an Island paradise for a break to one of Australia's most iconic holiday destinations. We decided to do this for numerous reasons. Hamilton Island is amazing but summer there is hot and tropical. The water in the sea or the swimming pools is warm and only just refreshing. There is no surf and the Iraganji jellyfish are a threat in the waters in the warmer weather. We didn't really feel like celebrating Christmas much either but the children deserved some sort of respite from this ongoing fight for Leah's life. We figured it would be more enjoyable without the constant reminders of home. We needed a break for the children from what Leah was going through. Maybe this would be her last Christmas with us. That was too much to contemplate. For the first time throughout Leah's illness I felt helpless. The Gold Coast offers beautiful sandy beaches, amazing surf and refreshing water. This would be a much deserved treat for the children. We had the use of a timeshare which I had bought many years ago and only used spasmodically. This was a good chance to use it. This meant the cost would be very little. This small Christmas holiday was a goal we could put some effort into that would take our minds off cancer for a while. But this would be only brief. We still had work to be done. Then something amazing happened.

While we were planning this trip for Christmas I was spending a bit of time on the internet. Booking trips, researching the Gold Coast and still looking at cancer information sites. One site that caught my eye was a site for Gamma Knife. I had never heard of it. I asked our doctors and not much information was known. I did some local searches but they all came up blank. I investigated more information and discovered that this treatment was developed in 1968 and they were improving it all the time. It was a version of stereotactic radiotherapy. I had heard of that. We had enquired about that earlier but they said it was not suitable. This looked different though. I don't know why but it sparked an interest so we made some enquiries. I did a search for an Australian centre offering this treatment. All the information was from overseas. The Australian Gamma Knife centre was actually in Hawaii. Why was that? I soon found out. Australia didn't have this technology but there was a significant demand for it so the clever people in Hawaii had decided to utilise this fact to fill the void. It was clever marketing. But as Gamma Knife was only available overseas it was also expensive. However it was Leah's life we were talking about so I sent off for some more information and was surprised by what came back. This technology was perfect for the exact cancer that Leah had. All of a sudden we were offered an option when we weren't offered anything in Australia. Australia had the Linear Accelerator which I mentioned earlier. This is similar technology but dated and less effective and as I indicated previously not of any use for Leah's situation. Finding out about the Linear Accelerator was such a long and tedious process and it was here in Australia. Yet we could find out about this Gamma Knife over night. We had sent Leah's scans to the doctor in Melbourne only for him to tell us that his Linear Accelerator was not an option for her. The Gamma Knife is different as it targets the tumours specifically using a head frame. It is very accurate. There would be little harm to surrounding tissue. Linear Accelerators are a bit more random. I was discovering that we were really a long way behind the rest of the world in cancer care yet it was such a high profile cause. We donate and spend billions each year but we lack so much. Why hadn't anyone told us about other options that are out there? Gamma Knife was a world recognised treatment but hardly anyone in Australia knew about it. I was baffled and quite frustrated by my discoveries. How many others were being denied world class treatment options?

We had a friend who lived in San Diego and this city had a Gamma Knife centre. So we enquired online and they gave us the instructions on how to determine if Gamma Knife was suitable for Leah. We had to forward Leah's patient history and her most recent scans. We had to post these as we didn't have them on a disk which we could have emailed to save time. But it only took a few days in the post. They then contacted us by email to give us the news that Leah was a suitable candidate. We were over the moon. Leah may not have received a miracle in India but was this a delayed miracle? Gamma Knife was used extensively throughout the world for exactly the type of cancer Leah now had. They were confident that this could help her. But it was expensive. It was over $20,000 US. With the exchange rate at the time this would make it about $38,000 in Australian dollars. But this was a small price to pay to save a human life. This was the woman I loved. It was for the children's mum. What would you do? We had both worked all of our lives so we had the ability to access money to pay for this upfront which was what was requested. No insurance would pay for this as we didn't live in America. We were going it alone. It was urgent for Leah to get the treatment so we just put it on our credit cards. No second thoughts what so ever. We would fix the monetary side of things up at a later stage. We needed to fix Leah first. It's funny how priorities change when faced with a life or death situation. If I was considering paying $30,000 for a new car or furniture I would have had butterflies or apprehension but this decision created none of those uncertainties. It just had to be done. After only a few days the treatment was organised. While in the USA Leah could stay at her friends. Gamma Knife only takes a day so it would only need to be a quick visit. Leah only had to get there.

We booked flights from Brisbane which is about an hour from the Gold Coast where we would be staying for Christmas. We had booked her flight to follow our Christmas holiday. As it was peak travel time the flight was expensive but it had to be done, we couldn't wait just to save a few dollars. Time was critical. These bloody tumours were growing as we waited. Soon the treatment was booked, flights were booked and all systems were go. Now it was time for a bit of a break. All this cancer business can be quite stressful. It was stressful for all of us. We went to the Gold Coast for our mini holiday. It was nice. This was a bit more celebratory than the last two times Leah, and myself in India, had been away. Those times we had been away from the family. As a family we celebrated Christmas on the Gold Coast and spent time at the beach and just relaxed. We were actually very relaxed as we now had a solution to Leah's health problems which had seemed quite remote only weeks before. The children wanted to visit the theme parks but with what we were paying out on Leah's treatment this could wait for next time. We just did the family things that you do at Christmas. The children still got presents and we ate and celebrated our unique family and our bizarre life. The Gold Coast was perfect for this. The weather was perfect and the surroundings were totally different to what we would have been experiencing back on Hamilton Island. The beaches are gorgeous with huge expanses of lovely white sand and the bluest water. We drove up into the Gold Coast hinterland on one of the days. We had a huge selection of cafes and restaurants to choose from and an amazing selection of the freshest fruit and vegetables to cook for our meals in our unit. A load had been taken off our minds and now we were really enjoying the holiday. After our family break on the Gold Coast we drove Leah to the airport in Brisbane. This was another awful drive. At the airport we had an emotional farewell but we knew Leah would be okay. This would be just another trip away from home. I don't know how Leah did it. She had faced death several times and now was flying into the unknown. Leah was flying off, alone. I would have given anything to have been able to accompany her but this was impossible due to the cost involved. That walk onto the plane for her must have been so frightening. Leah was off overseas and to what we hoped would be a life saving treatment. She assured us she would ring as soon as she got to the USA. Then she would have the treatment and before we knew it she would be home and getting better. The children were relieved knowing this information, especially about getting the phone call. They hated Leah being away but they did look forward to the phone calls. Leah then left, on her own, into the unknown. Why did she have to travel sixteen hours, overseas, for a treatment that had been available for many people worldwide for over thirty years? I was beginning to question our health care system in Australia. This trip was a daunting prospect for us at home. Leah, though, could only see the great outcome at the end of it all. She had been handed a potential lifeline when we could never have dreamed of one only weeks earlier. All the experts in Australia had drawn a blank but here was our miracle that we had been seeking. Leah was a pioneer.


Leah landed in LA and had to catch a train to San Diego. She was unable to make contact with her friend so decided she would just head off and stay in a hotel if need be in the meantime. She got to the station and only just made the train. She only just got on to the carriage and was all alone except for one other passenger. The other passenger was an 80 year old lady so Leah went over and sat near her. Her name was Jean. They struck up a conversation and Jean was shocked that Leah had to travel, on her own, half way around the world for her treatment. She was also not happy that Leah had not confirmed somewhere to stay.

Jean insisted that Leah come home and stay with her. So Leah did. No second thoughts. It just felt right. Was this lady an angel sent to look over Leah? Leah and Jean struck up an instant friendship. They got to know each other on the train trip to San Diego. Leah arrived at Jeans home just out of San Diego and felt right at home. It was a biggish house that Jean had to herself since her husband had died, a number of years earlier, so there was plenty of room. There were orange orchards outside so Jean would look after Leah and start her days with fresh juice. Jean helped Leah organise her appointments and Jean would ensure Leah got to those appointments as well. Leah required a pre treatment interview first of all. She met the doctors and other staff and instantly felt so confident in their abilities. It was very professional and very modern. They did a new round of scans as these were used to indicate to the doctors where the Gamma Knife would focus its treatment to kill the cancer yet not damage any healthy tissue of the brain. Jean would go in with Leah and stay with her until completion. Nothing was too much for her. She was such a generous person throughout the entire time Leah was with her. After the appointment with the doctors they would do a bit of sightseeing, visit some of Jean's friends, do some shopping, have cups of tea and talk about things Leah had not pondered as yet in her journey to date. When Leah rang to chat to us she was so excited, so positive and in a really happy place considering she was about to undergo brain cancer treatment. I could only sit back and admire the courage she had shown throughout her entire cancer battle. This new predicament was handled with strength, grace and courage. I did not feel worthy of such a woman in my life. I was truly blessed. We were both lucky Jean had been there for Leah. The following few days were taken up with more appointments to plan the treatment and explain it to Leah. The treatment, for nine brain tumours, would only take one day. In fact the entire treatment would take only a few hours. Leah felt so lucky to have Jean by her side all the way and she felt like she had the best medical care anyone in her situation could ask for. She was ready. She was looking forward to the future again. The children were excited. Leah was optimistic and full of hope and trust. It all felt right. These things happen for a reason. Jean was meant to be in Leah's life. Miracles were happening. This was an amazing twist to our seemingly helpless position of just a few weeks ago.

# Chapter 12

# Gamma Knife, A new beginning

Now Gamma Knife is not a knife at all. It is a funny name for this piece of equipment. We weren't overly concerned about the name. We were just hoping that it would get rid of the cancer whether that was by cutting it or blasting it out. Leah went in to the Gamma Knife centre on the morning after her scans had been analysed and the treatment plan created. They needed to attach a frame, which was like a massive motor cycle helmet with holes, to her skull. This was done with a cordless drill. It was drilled straight into her skull. I was shocked when I found this out. But it was the worst part of the whole ordeal. The rest was plain sailing. The frame would guide hundreds of beams to the exact spots in Leah's brain where the tumours were. It provided the accuracy and ensured no healthy tissue, skin or organs were damaged. Once the frame had been attached to Leah, she was put on to a trolley and this was fed into a chamber like an MRI machine. The frame was clipped in to place and kept still and the operators activated the beams which were guided through the frame and into the head but directed only at the cancer. This was truly amazing stuff. It was almost science fiction. Well it was for us. I was amazed that this type of thing had been around for decades yet we had never heard of it in Australia. I thought we were cancer treatment leaders but it appeared we weren't even cancer treatment followers. How many others were missing out on this option? How many families torn apart because of our lack of knowledge? Did we think we were so advanced that it was pride preventing us having this treatment in Australia? I hope this was not the case. I couldn't work out why countries such as India and Thailand had these treatments yet we didn't in Australia. The USA and Europe offered it but we didn't. But now we had found it and Leah was in the middle of seeing how it would all go. She said it was a bit claustrophobic but if that was the worst side effect of this treatment it was amazing. She meditated the entire time that she was being treated and before she knew it, the treatment was done. Her entire treatment was all over in a few short hours. Jean was there the entire time and was there to greet Leah when she emerged from the treatment room. Leah had little more than a slight headache. But this was expected after having a huge frame attached to your head and nine tumours being eradicated from her brain.

Leah said that the worst aspect of this treatment was having the frame, which was reasonably heavy, attached to her head and the fact she had to lie still for nearly three hours. Compared to what she had to endure for a month in Melbourne previously, this was a walk in the park. The frame was removed and Leah was ushered into a suite for recovery. She only needed an overnight stay. A bit of rest, some nourishment and then she could go home with Jean. Jean stayed at the hospital and made sure Leah was okay and then left her to rest only to return the next day to collect her.


Leah was not able to fly yet as there may be some swelling so she stayed with Jean some more until she was ready to return home. Qantas needed to get the all clear for her to travel. Most local patients would be able to go home to recover and return periodically for checkups but Leah only had Jean and then, after the airline had given the approval for Leah to travel, she would return to Australia. Leah had a phone card so kept in contact with us and the children were so happy to have the daily chats with their mum. I was just so excited that Jean had been so helpful, supportive and generous. She truly was a marvel. It was lovely to be able to share this fantastic story of Leah's guardian angel with the children. It took away a lot of the concern the children were having with mum being alone and on the other side of the world.

Leah went in for follow up visits and all looked well. The actual procedure had been administered successfully. The proof would be in the pudding. But we wouldn't know for a while. Long after Leah would have returned to Australia. This wasn't a perfect situation as the doctors who had looked after her in San Diego would not be able to take much of a role in her progress due to the distance Leah would be from them. But it's a smaller world these days and we could use things like email to keep tabs on Leah's progress once she returned home. However before Leah came back to Australia she was able to enjoy a few more days with Jean. This was a far cry from Leah's experience after the less than successful radiation treatment she had endured in Australia previously. She had no ability or energy after that for anything and required many drugs just to counter the side effects. It was a different story in San Diego. Jean took Leah to her local church service. They did some sightseeing. They indulged in some shopping. They both prepared healthy meals for themselves and some of Leah's new friends. Leah really enjoyed the experience of the last few days with Jean. She reflected on her luck in finding this brilliant treatment. She had been given a second chance and was extremely grateful for that opportunity. She had enjoyed the new start to her new life and Jean had been a wonderful introduction to this. Once

Leah had recovered and the airline gave her approval to travel it was time to come home. It was a bitter sweet moment. She had met a wonderful new friend in Jean. She had experienced world class cancer care administered by such compassionate and professional staff. But she also couldn't wait to get home to us.

Our neighbour was the minister on Hamilton Island. Non denominational, he catered for all. There was a lovely chapel just near us where he would conduct weddings and church services on a Sunday. Leah attended the church services on most of the times they ran. I would take the children sometimes but they either got a bit bored or Leah wanted this experience as private time. So the children didn't attend that often. Terry would finish the service by reading a children's book. They always had a moral to the story. When I attended Terry's services I would leave in tears as these books really had an emotional effect. This started a love of quality children's books which remains with our family today. Terry also took a great interest in me. He would drag me away for a coffee from time to time. He would check on how I was doing. He wanted to give me some away time. He offered me some nurturing and counseling. Terry is a wise and very generous man. He is gentle and supportive. He did a lot for many people on and off Hamilton Island but the times he spent checking on me were very much appreciated and still move me today. I had been lucky to meet some truly amazing people in my life and Terry and his wife Amanda were two of the best. He also, unknowingly, helped Leah deal with many issues during her illness. The children's books were part of that. While Leah was in USA she shopped for really special gifts to bring back for the children. A couple of these were children's books with such special meaning. Just prior to Leah leaving for Australia, she and Jean did a bit of shopping to fill in the time and fulfill Leah's desire for some special mementos to bring home. How amazing is it that after treatment for nine brain tumours she was able to go shopping. One of the books she purchased, which would have a huge effect on all of our lives, was by famous actor Jamie Lee Curtis. It was a kids book, beautifully written and illustrated called "I'm gonna like me". It is all about self esteem and liking yourself for you not what others think. It was a well timed purchase due to the stage of life our children were in. Bec was entering her teens and Bim had already endured so much in his short life so far. The book was a timely reminder to us all about the important things in life.

The other book Leah brought back was called "The next place" and was about death and what happens after. It was a children's book but had such a universal message that I dare anyone to read it and not be moved. We had never mentioned the possibility of Leah's death but while alone overseas she had contemplated the possibility and faced it. She bought the books to help us deal with what could lie ahead - who knew? These two books were purchased and set Leah up for the unknown but helped her face any uncertainties with confidence. She wanted to ensure the children were strong and that they understood what may happen in the future. It was the first time, I am aware of, that Leah had faced these thoughts. It was a sad time as she had not allowed these thoughts to be publicly aired previously. She tried to avoid them to ensure she remained strong to enhance her ability to stay healthy. Having the time away, meeting new people and experiencing new technologies enabled Leah to welcome these thoughts and the strength they gave her to carry on. It took a lot of the worry about us, the children and I, away and allowed her to focus on getting better. She had been through so much in a few short years but it was a couple of children's books that helped her move forward. The books were also an informative and non confronting means in which we could explain things to the children. The children had obviously experienced the physical signs of Leah's cancer journey but the specifics of what was going on were quite often missed by them. This experience with the Gamma Knife,

San Diego and Jean was a conduit to enabling them to understand more of what had happened with Leah and what could happen in the future. We all grew quite significantly during this time.

The enormity of Leah's journey to San Diego had not gone unnoticed in the USA. An Aussie mum having to travel to the other side of the globe for cancer treatment. The staff at the hospital laughed at this fact in amazement. But there was also huge admiration of the tenacity of this spunky Aussie chick. They may have thought that Australia really was a backwater with kangaroos bouncing down the main street. But it was an amazing story. Someone tipped off a journalist at the San Diego Tribune and they wanted to do a story. Diane Bell came and interviewed both Jean and Leah. The background, the discovery of this treatment, the trip, the chance meeting on the train, the support Jean had offered, the friendship, the trust and the family left behind thousands of miles away. They took a photo and the story ran while Leah was still in San Diego. It was titled "Never take in a stranger - Well it can be inspiring." The story of an 80 year old local woman who did take in a stranger and helped her cope during an extremely unknown and totally frightening experience without a second thought and with so much care and generosity. Leah and her family back home could never thank Jean enough for what she did. Or could they?

The Gamma Knife centre where Leah had her treatment decided they would run a similar story in their newsletter. It had a bit more on the treatment side of things but also included the human interest angle as well because this helped show the journey with cancer in a far more positive way. Leah decided then and there to ensure that Australians should not have to endure the emotions and expense that she had and that she would raise awareness of this treatment when she returned. That return would not be far away now as she had recovered enough to be okay to fly. Most people having Gamma Knife don't need as much recovery time. However due to the number of tumours and also her need to fly at the conclusion of the treatment, a slightly longer recovery period was needed. Leah had spent a few more days at Jeans house after leaving hospital but the entire time in the USA was only ten days. Only one day for the treatment. Most of her time was spent shopping, sightseeing and meeting new friends. This was cancer treatment as we'd never seen before.

# Chapter 13

# Home Sweet Home. Now to pay for it all

I was very nervous about Leah coming home. Last time, when she returned from the treatment in Melbourne, had been very difficult to cope with. It had a bad effect on the children to see their mum in such bad shape. It had taken Leah so long to get over that experience as well. The kids had never seen her that bad. I had never seen her that bad. But hopefully this time would be much better. It was now a new year and we had enjoyed our break away at the Gold Coast. I also hoped Leah had enjoyed San Diego even given the circumstances of the trip. We had spoken nearly every day and heard all about Jean and the amazing facility that offered the Gamma Knife. The tone of our communication was now so much more positive since finding out about the Gamma Knife. We couldn't wait to be together again. I had missed her so much. One of the biggest impacts cancer had made in our lives was the amount of time spent away from each other. The time had come on this occasion though for Leah to return. Leah was due home so we went to the airport to greet her. She had flown in to Sydney initially and then boarded a connecting flight to Hamilton Island. It took about twenty hours. This was not the ideal conclusion to a pretty major procedure on a person's brain. We were at the airport waiting when she arrived. It was amazing. She looked fantastic. She had a couple of little indentations where they had inserted the screws to attach the Gamma Knife frame to her skull but apart from that she looked sensational, was in extremely high spirits and was healthy and vibrant. We all hugged her and the relief in seeing Leah so well was obvious. We got in the buggy and went home. This was a totally different experience to her arrival home from Melbourne after her whole head radiation. Last time the children were afraid to touch her. She had looked different after being away for over a month on that occasion. She was also very fragile that time. This time the children swamped her and helped Leah unpack knowing that many treats would be on offer. They were right. Leah had brochures, photos, books and fond memories of a previously unknown treatment and a daunting journey. It had been expensive. Treatment, scans, hospital stays, airfares, transfers and incidentals but every penny was well spent when we looked at the result. We had mum back. We had discovered something by accident. We knew nothing about it. Leah's doctors in Australia could offer very little information about it. Leah had travelled half way around the world into the unknown. She had returned as good as new. We had taken a risk but it was definitely worth every doubt, every cent and every hurdle to achieve. This again was miraculous. Our miracle had come quite some time after our trip to India. But at least it had come.


It truly was sensational how good Leah looked. She would now start campaigning to get this treatment to Australia as she was so impressed with it. Who wouldn't be? She was almost killed by the only treatment offered in Australia, which had failed to do anything to the nasty cancer in her head. Now after basically one day of treatment she was back to her old self. Leah was busting with excitement. She needed to tell people about this experience. People deserved to know about the Gamma Knife. She contacted newspapers, television shows and hospitals to tell them of her experience. Leah's oncologist in Melbourne was so impressed with her results he used her experience in a presentation he was doing in Switzerland. We asked him why he hadn't mentioned this treatment to us and he explained that as we didn't have it in Australia most doctors weren't informed enough of Gamma Knife's capabilities. This was partly due to the lack of opportunity to learn about it. It was also due to relevance. It seemed pointless doing much research as we didn't have Gamma Knife in Australia to use the knowledge afterwards anyway. As oncologists and doctors were so busy with other treatments being used, their focus was on researching products being introduced or used in Australia. As most of these were drugs that were being offered a lot of research or knowledge had to be gained into suitability of these products and the side effects. We were amazed at the lack of knowledge in regard to other options that should be available or at least mentioned in discussions with someone dealing with cancer. Especially someone who has been given no treatment options and basically been told to prepare for a quick death. Leah's oncologist also mentioned that he didn't recommend Gamma Knife due to the cost. We thought this was just so wrong as it should be up to the recipient to determine if they could afford it or not. So armed with all this information about Gamma Knife and firsthand experience Leah began her quest.  It was a quest to help others receive better options in cancer care in Australia. People would ask a number of questions during this time. One was the cost. Leah felt that the cost was irrelevant in the scheme of things and the cost should not be a reason for not mentioning potential lifesaving treatments. The other thing she had found was that when she came back from her treatment in Melbourne Leah was unable to work for months. This resulted in severe loss of income. After the Gamma Knife she was able to commence work virtually straight away. After her jet lag had subsided anyway. So the actual cost involved by having Gamma Knife was offset by things such as ability to work and quality of life. Now that I have mentioned the affordability of Gamma Knife I will progress on to how we were going to pay for it. Well we had already paid for it but that was on credit at high interest. In just a few days since returning from the USA Leah felt well enough to work. So she did. I worked in the Human Resources department and we needed a recruitment coordinator. Leah applied and even though she had no experience in this field, she got the job. A bit of basic training and she was ready. It was an office job and we felt it suited our needs better at the moment. It sure beat the shift work of her previous role. Leah was still doing meditation and all the other activities to ensure her good health and this job offered set hours so Leah could maintain her health improvement activities. Leah's parents gave us some money for the treatment which we paid straight off the debt. Leah was thankful for this but we paid that back as soon as we could as well. Leah's parents were getting older and they needed the money so we made it a priority to pay that back. As we had both been working for most of the time Leah had been battling cancer it was quite easy to get into the routine of budgeting to pay off this debt. Unfortunately Leah still required regular scans to track the progress of the tumours. The costs of travel and the scans ate into our funds and it was taking ages to get anywhere. But we were used to the costs associated with cancer so it was just part of our lives now. Money would come in and money would go out. Just at different times it was at different rates.

# A surprise would be nice.

Life was pretty good. Leah was fit and healthy again. She began working again so quickly after her brain cancer treatment. The children were happy. They had their fit, vibrant, healthy mum back.  We lived in paradise. Could it get any better? Of course it could. We got some great news. Eighty year old Jean from San Diego was going to pay us a visit. She had never even been to the movies on her own and here she was travelling half way around the world, on her own, to come for a visit. We decided that we would pay for her accommodation at the Beach Club which is where Leah used to work. It was the best choice of accommodation at the resort at the time. Jean would stay with us for about a week and then visit the Northern Territory and see Uluru. Then she would continue on to Melbourne to meet and visit Leah's parents. We were so excited. We had heard all about Jean but not actually met her. It was an opportunity to say a huge thank you to her for looking after Leah when she was in the USA getting her Gamma Knife treatment.

The day arrived. Leah met Jean at the airport and she brought her home in the golf buggy. Jean loved it. It was such a unique setting for her to experience. The children had drawn a huge welcome sign and picture, with chalk, on our driveway. Jean was welcomed by this and the two very excited children upon her arrival at our unit. Jean came bearing gifts for the children. It was an emotional time. We found it very exciting but also a time of reflection, awe and gratitude. Jean was lovely. We spent the week with Jean doing all the touristy stuff. Leah and Jean snorkeled on the Great Barrier Reef. They went to the mainland for Leah's check up and Jean went along to see some of rural Australia which included the cane fields. We had an attraction on Hamilton Island called Safari tours. A four wheel drive truck that takes guests to a secluded beach for an Aussie BBQ dinner, guitar music and didgeridoo. This was very Australian and Jean really enjoyed it. She even had a go at the didgeridoo. This was a very naughty thing for a female to do in Aboriginal customs but she was 80 years of age. She wasn't scared of the ramifications. The Safari tour was always a favourite. It was a great thing for the children as well. Jean also got to pat and hold the koalas at the Koala Gallery the next morning. We always took visitors to this little attraction which featured a lovely breakfast and lots of animals to look at. You could also have a hold of a koala or crocodile and have your photo taken. Jean opted for the koala option. It was not all fun and frivolity. We had an unexpected and quite amazing thing happen during Jeans visit as well. The local newspaper, The Whitsunday Times, had heard of her visit and wanted to do a story on Leah and Jean. They had both been in the San Diego news while Leah was there and now Jean would be in our news. This was an amazing situation and Jean just loved it. The week flew by but it was also filled with some wonderful memories. Jean became part of our family. We could see why Leah didn't hesitate to trust Jean on the train in California. She was awesome. We all loved her and everyone who met her and heard the story just felt the same way. She loved Australia and the people. The trip had been a real winner. I couldn't thank her enough. It was like she was my grandmother and I had been a part of her family all my life. Such was the bond formed by her generosity and genuine care for my wife and now our entire family. But the time soon came to an end. Jean had to leave. It was sad to see her go but we knew she would just love the rest of the trip. Going to Melbourne would give Leah's parents a chance to thank Jean as well. Jean's time in the red centre of Australia would also be a great experience for her. After her whirlwind tour of our vast country Jean was soon back in the USA but we had forged a lifelong bond with her as she had also done with Leah's parents.

Leah was determined now to get Gamma Knife to Australia. She spent a vast amount of time writing, petitioning and talking to as many people as possible. The people who had seen the change in her after just one day of treatment were amazed. She wrote to television programs, newspapers, magazines and politicians. No takers. She contacted medical professionals, hospitals and local government but no one listened or showed any interest. How could we discover such a breakthrough and have it ignored? This made no sense. Then something strange happened. The Australian cricket team came to Hamilton Island for a break after a season of games. Jane McGrath was the wife of legend fast bowler Glenn. I saw Glenn at the bar and when I saw Leah later I informed her of this. Jane, his wife, was a high profile breast cancer patient. We had read the McGrath's book earlier on in Leah's journey with cancer. Leah was excited by the prospect of getting someone famous to assist her getting a great cancer treatment to Australia. Leah rang the hotel reception and asked to speak to Jane. Jane and Tracey Bevan, who was cricketer Michael's wife, ran the McGrath Foundation. This wonderful foundation was raising much needed funds and awareness for breast cancer. They were wonderful on the phone with Leah and agreed to meet with her. They popped over to have afternoon tea with Leah at our unit and discuss Gamma Knife. Jane's idea for her foundation was to fund breast cancer nurses. This would mean that a patient would go to hospital with breast cancer and had the same or at least a specialist breast cancer nurse throughout their treatment journey. Tracey and Jane thought Gamma Knife sounded great but as it was a brain cancer treatment it didn't fit into the McGrath foundations vision. But they said they would make some enquiries to see if someone else could run with it. Leah also explained that she was a breast cancer patient initially. She had met many breast cancer patients who were now battling cancer in a different part of their bodies. Leah's secondary cancer just happened to be in the brain. This thing, unfortunately, happened quite a lot and Leah wanted to help other breast cancer survivors' battle secondary cancer if it eventuated. However Jane and Tracey felt they were unable to help. Leah was disappointed. Even though the afternoon was less than fruitful, in regard to Gamma Knife, it was still enjoyable to meet two such amazing woman doing remarkable things. They were high profile people but also great friends and they were making a difference. This was truly inspiring and extremely encouraging for Leah and myself. However the next few months were frustrating for Leah. She had stumbled upon this great treatment that had been around for thirty years and could help so many in Australia but it all fell on deaf ears. She needed a break.

# Chapter 14

# Field of women, Good Morning Australia, Bert, Patti and Marcia

Leah was asked, by her friend in Melbourne, to join her at the Field of Women event at the MCG. This is an event put on by the breast cancer network to raise money and awareness for breast cancer. Thousands of women turn up at the Melbourne Cricket Ground, which holds 100,000 people, prior to a Friday evening Aussie rules football match. They don pink ponchos as a symbol of defiance against cancer and to show support to people battling cancer, or who have battled it and won or people who have lost the fight. Joy, Leah's friend, had lived on Hamilton Island before us and we had consulted with her before moving there ourselves. Joy had been sick with Non Hodgkins Lymphoma and it was an ironic battle that she shared with Leah. When Joy was well, Leah would be sick and vice versa. Joy had been sick on Hamilton Island and due to this didn't have as much of a time to enjoy it as we had. She now lived in Melbourne and this is why Leah agreed to go to the Field of Women. Leah had to go to Melbourne for her regular scans and to visit her oncologist anyway. This allowed Leah to fit in a dinner with Joy and then visit the Field of Women. We were able to see some news flashes on television as it is a huge event Australia wide. Leah and Joy went and participated in this glorious celebration of people affected in so many ways by breast cancer. They met Raelene Boyle who is a famous Australian athlete who had battled breast cancer and beaten it. Leah also spied Lauren Newton who is the daughter of an iconic Australian couple, Bert and Patti Newton. This legendary couple had, at the time, a national morning show on the television and had done decades of amazing variety shows as well. Bert's current show was called Good Morning Australia. Lauren was guest reporting for the network and doing interviews and commentaries on the Field of Women event. Leah told Joy she was going to get interviewed by Lauren and discuss the Gamma Knife. If you knew Leah you would know of her determination. If she set her mind to something it usually came to fruition. Getting interviewed by Lauren was going to happen. And it did. Now as a result of that interview Patti Newton decided she would have Leah come on to the show and do an interview with Patti and her husband Bert. So the journey to Melbourne was enjoyable for Leah and had been a huge success in her determination to spread awareness of the Gamma Knife. She returned home to us extremely happy and excited. But she would soon be going away again. But this time it was for a positive reason. We didn't mind her going away this time. Leah was fit and healthy and wanted to share all the information she had with the world. Bert's television show was a start and quite a significant one. As we lived on Hamilton Island they had to fly Leah back to Melbourne for the show. Another trip away but it was paid for this time. This was one of the biggest changes in our lives regarding this rotten cancer. There was so much travel involved. The time away was hard for all of us. It was difficult for the children. But the reason for the travel lately was good rather than bad. Leah was used to travelling for a treatment or a chance at getting better. This trip to Melbourne was a chance for Leah to give back. It was an opportunity for Leah to help others. She had received so much support over the years that she felt obliged to help by raising awareness of the Gamma Knife. They did fly her to Melbourne and she stayed overnight and caught up with friends and family. On the day of the interview she went to the television station, had her makeup done and waited in the green room with Marcia Hines. Marcia is an Australian legend of music that had come to live in Australia from USA many decades before. She had been the Queen of pop, been in award winning shows and had dozens of albums to her name. After chatting in the green room, Marcia invited Leah to her show at the Crown casino that night. When I heard this story I was in awe of what Leah had achieved. After her chat with Marcia Hines it was Leah's turn to be interviewed. She did so well. I was so proud of her. Bert and Patti were warm, funny and genuinely interested in Leah's amazing story. We watched on the television from Hamilton Island. Bert and Patti asked questions about Leah's journey, they flashed photo's up on the screen of all of us and we got mentions. Hamilton Island also got mentioned. The kids and the school got mentioned. Even Jean from San Diego got a mention. Then they moved on to the Gamma Knife. They explained the process, where it could be accessed and asked Leah of her experience and success. They showed images of Leah getting the treatment in USA. Then they commented on the Field of Women event where all this had started. It was a lengthy and informative interview. Leah was very nervous and Patti alluded to a saying Leah loved to say. However with the pressure of the cameras Leah got a bit confused and Patti had to help but she got it out in the end. It went something like this and Leah loved saying it to others.

Yesterday's history

Tomorrows a mystery

Today is the present

That's why it's called a gift


Leah rang as soon as the segment was all finished. She was ecstatic. She said Bert and Patti were so funny, natural and warm during the entire show. Leah had publicly started her campaign for better cancer care options in Australia and now felt she could make a difference. She already had. We were inundated with phone calls from people all over the country so excited at seeing Leah on television. They were so proud of her courage. Courage in the way she had fought cancer so fiercely and proud that she was now trying to help others. Leah was paving the way to better cancer care in Australia.

That night Leah caught up with her friend Megan. Megan is a bit of a celebrity in Melbourne. Her celebrity status started slowly but grew to become one of the biggest profiles in Australia at one stage. Years after this evening with Leah and as a result of Leah's belief in positive affirmations, that Megan also followed, Megan would meet Oprah Winfrey and then have dinner with Oprah when she visited Melbourne. Leah's cancer story gets more amazing every day. Who would have thought it would now have Oprah in it? Leah's friend Megan makes amazing jewelry. She also had a bed linen range in department stores and we even have a couple of photo albums she designed and sold in huge retail outlets. It is her jewelry, though, that she was most proud of and that she is known for. She was always in the celebrity pages in the news and she really is an amazing woman. Megan is very social but extremely generous in action and thought. She could be forgiven for being too busy for all her friends but she somehow finds the time. Megan took Leah to see Marcia Hines in concert that evening, after the television interview. It was a great ending to an eventful few days and was a chance for Leah to relax. At the show, Marcia knew that Leah was in the audience. She explained to the crowd how they met and of Leah's journey and asked if the audience would mind if she sang a song to Leah and for Leah. Of course the audience loved it. However the band didn't know of this and hadn't rehearsed for it. So Marcia sang the song called "From the inside" acapella style. This famous song features the line "Come on girl, you can do it". Well, from all accounts, there wasn't a dry eye in the house. This song became a bit of a theme song for Leah after that night. Leah's life had been full of twists and turns but some of the stories in it are just too good to keep to ourselves. This was one of those times. She had achieved what she had set out to do. Her adventure in Melbourne, the television show and the concert were just reward for someone who had been through so much. She was then finished with Melbourne for the moment and returned to us. When Leah left Melbourne she received a package. It was a thank you from Bert and Patti. The package had vouchers for flights to Melbourne, a hotel stay for the gorgeous Como hotel and a three course dinner at a restaurant across the road from the Como. Upon returning to Hamilton Island Leah showed me this lovely gift and we were excited to be able to plan to use it very soon. We had all been through so much, worked so hard and missed our family being together. This lovely touch from Bert and Patti was welcomed with open arms. We took the trip to Melbourne very soon after Leah returned. We took the children with us and they stayed with their grandparents and Leah and I went and had a lovely romantic dinner and luxury hotel stay. We hadn't had much to celebrate until recently. Nor did we have the finances now to be able to do something as extravagant as this. Everything was perfect and as Leah's health was so good we let our hair down and indulged. We had a few drinks. Leah had a steak which she didn't do a great deal anymore as she had virtually been vegetarian for ages. We even had dessert. The next morning we had a lovely breakfast that was included and our indulgent stay at the Como was complete. I still have the rubber duck that was placed in the gorgeous bathroom as a unique touch by the hotel. It was nice to be like a normal couple for a change, doing what many couples do on special occasions. It had been a romantic date. It was some quality time by ourselves and we laughed and had fun. We were able to block out any bad elements of our lives for a time and just enjoy the experience and each other. I hadn't been to Melbourne for some time so this was an extra special treat for me. Leah had been on her own several times but not for leisure. This was the perfect surprise given to us by Bert and Patti.

It had been a very generous action by the people at Good Morning Australia so when we returned to Hamilton Island Leah contacted the producers to pass on our sincere gratitude. While they were talking they had an idea. They would send a film crew up and we could record a thank you on camera to be televised on the show. As Bert had mentioned the children on the segment with Leah, they decided to include the children and the school. I was at work on the day they came up but the cameras went to the school and they filmed Leah saying a big thankyou to Bert. They then panned to all the school children who all yelled out hi as well. Of course our 2 kids were closest to the camera. This was a fitting finale to an amazing experience for Leah and the message was out about the other options for cancer treatment that most Australians are still, even today, not aware of. I added a video of Leah's adventures on Good Morning Australia on to the Facebook site called Elvis, Dirty dancing and a tornado or 2, if you would like to see it for yourself. This site was set up as an information site for this book and also to update everyone on the books progress. We had been through a lot. I wanted people to be able to share the experiences. Leah did as well.

**Leah always said that if this process helped save one life it would be a job well done. I liked the sound of that.**

# Chapter 15

# Leaving one paradise for a new paradise

The Gamma Knife had enabled Leah to achieve so much more than she was expected to be able to. Many months earlier she was given the worst news possible. But now she had seen Bim's first day of school and how lucky was he to be able to share that with his sister who was in year six at the same school. What an experience for the children to be able to attend school on a tropical island in paradise. Heading overseas for Gamma Knife had also allowed Leah to meet Jean and strike up an amazing friendship with her. Leah had now also been on the television numerous times. She had returned to work and was as vibrant as I'd seen her in ages. Things were certainly looking rosy at that time. However we had some big decisions to make as well. Rebecca would be beginning high school the following year. If she went to school on the mainland across from Hamilton Island it would mean a 7am start to catch the ferry. Bec would have to catch a connecting bus to get to school and then the same trek on the way home. This would mean she would not get home until after 5 pm. We weren't sure of the school either so we felt this was not an option. Mackay had a boarding school where students stay during the week and then go home for weekends. Rebecca loved that idea. Leah hated it. So that option was off the list. She could board full time in Brisbane. Some friends had done that with their children and it worked really well and the kids were very well educated and just lovely people. However this would mean we would hardly see Bec so it was a big no again. We, especially Leah, had missed so much of the children so she didn't want to send Bec away and miss any more. This was going to take a lot of thinking and investigating. We were used to this type of research as we had done it so often in the past. This was more pleasant thought than researching cancer care alternatives. We then thought of an option that had presented itself to us but we weren't aware of it at the time. While we had been on holiday, last year, on the Gold Coast, before Leah's journey to the USA, we caught up with a few friends at Lennox Heads. This is a lovely town on the far North Coast of NSW. While on the Gold Coast we had taken the short trip to Byron Bay for a look at this stunning part of Australia. We had then travelled the short distance to our friend's house at Lennox Heads. We had a lovely day there and Pauline, who had come on our honeymoon, had come up from Melbourne to meet us as well. When it was time to go we decided not to go through Byron Bay again as it was so busy. It was Christmas holidays and Byron Bay was extremely busy and the traffic was at a standstill. Byron Bay is stunning, has beautiful beaches and an extremely laid back lifestyle so it is a popular holiday destination for Australians and people from overseas. As it is a little country seaside town it gets very congested during peak times. It only has one road in and one road out. This is why we had decided not to go back the same way we had driven earlier. So we went inland a bit and discovered a wonderful part of Australia known as the Byron hinterland. This was absolutely stunning. It was less built up than the seaside villages and towns. This journey took us through beautiful lush hills, quaint villages and miles of rain forest. This was heaven. It was an absolute paradise. We felt like we were in the Garden of Eden. I hope you get the idea. It was stunning. Yet we never thought of it as a potential home. We just loved the drive back to the Gold Coast at the time.

But looking at schooling options for Rebecca we thought back to that part of the trip. It had slipped our minds due to the main focus of that trip at Christmas, which was getting Leah off safely to America. Now we thought it might shape part of our future. We began to make it happen. I arranged to get the Byron Shire Echo sent up each week in the post. The Echo was the local paper of the Byron region and contained everything we needed to learn about the area. We got to know a lot about Byron Bay and the small towns around it. The newspaper had a classifieds section and we researched this wonderful part of the world. The Byron region had two Steiner schools and we thought this might be more suitable for Rebecca as she was more artistically inclined than academic. This was beginning to take shape. The Steiner school seemed amazing. We decided that this would be Rebecca's next school. We had made the decision. With the school sorted we looked at some rental properties in the paper. There were quite a few. We decided that we needed to nurture Leah's being. So with this in mind we researched small acreage properties. Neither of us had ever lived on the land but we thought it would be ideal for Leah and a fantastic experience for the children. The Byron area is well known for its beautiful environment, organic produce, fresh water and serenity. This would help us all. We could get back to nature. We would be surrounded by peace and quiet. In the end we didn't know if we'd cope with this but it was worth a try. We decided to rent first to make sure it was what we really wanted for the long term. We found a place in the newspaper and enquired. It was available and sounded perfect for what we wanted in our new life. So we took it. Sight unseen. It was all organised quite quickly. This was midyear. Leah had been really well for over six months now. We had just made the decision to move forward with our lives. We had organised a new place to live. We had started to arrange the next step for the children. Bec could start high school in the new year but both the kids would need to attend 1 semester of primary school first. It was all falling in to place. We were going. We were leaving one paradise to go and live in a new paradise. We had left the suburbs 18 months ago and now we could never go back. Life was good again. We left Hamilton Island and all of our wonderful friends the day after the Island Kindy Ball. The Kindy Ball was a once a year social event not to be missed. It was held in the Convention centre on Hamilton Island. At the time this Convention centre was the second largest one in Queensland. This gives you an idea of the size of this event. There was ample food, drinks, dancing and lots of fun. This was a huge night that was all for a good cause. The main focus was to raise money for the Island Kindy. The staff at the Kindy did a great job looking after our kids while they were young and while they were not quite old enough to start school. Everyone on Hamilton Island looked forward to this night of nights. This was definitely not the best night to follow up with an early start the next morning. However we did have a very early start and a long trek in our little blue car. The Kindy Ball was huge. It was a great night and a fitting finale to our wonderful time on Hamilton Island. The Ball was also a great event that got everyone together so this was a fantastic night to say our goodbyes. It was also a late night. We enjoyed it but it was bitter sweet. It was great to catch up with everyone. We got to dance and have so much fun. But during the night there were lots of tears as well.

We were a bit fuzzy in the morning but we were organised. Our furniture had gone and we were about to go to as well.

All our friends turned up at the ferry terminal to send us off in style and make it an extremely emotional event. We had some wonderful memories here in this tropical paradise. We had a few scares as well. We were leaving but we would never forget. We had made lifelong friends. Our lives were about to change again but these memories would remain.

We decided to not go to our new home straight away but head further north to see Bowen, Townsville, Cairns, Port Douglas, Cape Tribulation and then, after we had seen all this, we could travel to back down to Northern NSW and our new life. As Australia is such a big country we decided to see the tropical far North of Queensland at this time, while we had the chance, as we may never have the opportunity again. We had a lovely time and cancer was nowhere to be seen or heard. It was a lovely trip. The far North of Queensland is stunning. It is a unique part of the country. We loved the tropics, the relaxed pace and the sites we had heard so much of but never seen before. It was a nice treat for the whole family and a break for the children before they started their new life, school and social experiences. We took our time. We enjoyed the lack of pressure to be anywhere on time. We were in our little blue Festiva so we really had no choice. We visited glorious gorges. We went to beachside markets. We wandered through the streets of Cairns. We picked fruit off the tree. We ate ice cream made from the fruit grown nearby. The children swam. We hiked. We had afternoon tea in the rainforest. We took a chairlift over the rainforest canopy. We took a wonderful little train up a mountain. We travelled on boats past huge crocodiles. We drove through little villages which were off the beaten track. Many of our recent experiences were tinged with fear. This was an amazing break filled with joy and no fears. It was the perfect break between our two paradise homes. Once we finished exploring this lovely part of the world it was time to turn around and head south to our new home. It took four days to drive from the tropical North of Queensland to the sub tropical north of NSW. We were in no hurry. But at the same time we were excited to see our new home for the first time.

Our new home was at a place called Rosebank. It was about 20 minutes from Byron Bay. It was on ten acres. It had a stream meandering through the property. We also had beautiful rainforest surroundings. We had a general store about two kilometres away. We could walk to the store, grab a great coffee, which was grown just around the corner and walk home. It was a fantastic place to get some locally grown fruit, a carton of milk and it was the post office as well. It had a great little café next to it to. We would often go to Lismore which was 15 minutes further inland. Lismore had an organic market, farmers market and general facilities that you would find in quite a large town. There was a hospital in Lismore which Leah quickly became acquainted with. The children still had one semester of school to complete and the Rosebank school was just up the road and the bus stopped at our driveway to pick them up each morning and drop them off in the afternoon. Rebecca was still in Year six and Bim was in Kindy, so they got to help each other out, make new friends and get in to the swing of the new school together. It was a great school with only fifty children and a great principal and lovely teachers. Leah and I quickly got in to the great lifestyle this region offered. We would wake with the sun coming up. The front verandah was a great space to meditate and feel the gentle sun on our faces. We could grow or purchase fantastic fresh food for meals and juices. We explored. We made new friends. We loved everything about the new environment. It was relaxing and healthy. It was a great environment for the children. The great open spaces for them to explore and new friendships to develop. We had no television either. We loved our new life. We had made another fantastic decision. Once we were settled we rang a friend in Melbourne, Pauline, who we had been on our honeymoon with. She asked where we were living. She knew Rosebank. A friend of hers, who Leah knew of, lived just around the corner. Pauline's other friend, Jenny, was the one we visited at Christmas, at Lennox Heads, which gave us the introduction to this area and made us want to move here in the first instance. It was great that we had mutual friends straight away. This made us feel at home. Pauline's friend Jacinta lived about three kilometres away. We walked around one afternoon to introduce ourselves. Jacinta is married to Simon. They have two daughters. One was Rebecca's age and the other a bit older. They were both lovely girls. Even Bim loved this family. It was really comforting to have these guys just around the corner from us. We would have dinner with Simon and Jacinta on a regular basis. Leah would wander around to their house and do mosaic work on the verandah with Jacinta. Life was really nice at Rosebank. I planted a huge array of vegetables and flowering plants. The climate was unbelievably good for growing things. It was a sub tropical environment with plenty of heat and water. The experiment of moving to Rosebank was a success. We wanted it to be permanent. We also had to look ahead to Rebecca's school for next year. This was to be her first at high school. Mullumbimby, which was about twenty minutes away, had the Steiner school. We were going to send Bec to this school. So we decided this would be the place to move to permanently and we began looking for suitable houses to purchase. I had been working at a lovely cafe in the gorgeous town of Bangalow. The cafe was only open during the day and it was great to get back into the hospitality caper at an operational level. Neither of us had worked in a few months so it helped with the saving (or should that be medical debt reduction?) Our immediate life was great and our future was beginning to fall into place. We bought an old 1972 Datsun ute which we had grand plans of using to take to the markets and we were working on what we could sell at the markets. This was a real change of pace and lifestyle. We actually did a market stall and loaded the ute up with a couple of hay bales and we put a Cruel Sea CD in the player to create atmosphere. We sold Rocky Road in little Asian take away boxes. It was a huge success. We now had some direction for the future as well. A few months later we bought a house on ten acres at Wilsons Creek which is about five minutes from Mullumbimby. It was a real fixer upper but we had the money coming in and planned to do a renovation. We had also just sold our house in Melbourne and that helped with the purchase. The children finished that year at Rosebank and the plan was for Rebecca to go to the Steiner school and Bim would go to the local Wilsons Creek school. This was a lovely school which was close by and still only had about 50 students. The wife of the principal from Rosebank worked at the Wilsons Creek School. This was all falling into place. We moved to Wilsons Creek just before Christmas. We had family and friends from all over Australia come up for our first Christmas in our new home. We hadn't started the renovation yet but we would just after Christmas. Our new life was progressing nicely.

# Chapter 16

# Oh no, not again

The new year began quite slowly for us. Our visitors had gone. We could begin planning. I was working and we were to begin the renovation. The idea was to knock out the walls of four little rooms to open the house up and make a bigger, light filled living space. We arranged all of this and it was really nice to have a project to focus on and take our minds off the things of the past few years. It was great to focus on positive things and to look to our future together. Our renovation was a way of helping us build that new future. Leah was well and got to have a brilliant Christmas with friends and relatives and she got to enjoy the holidays with the children. Soon, though, it was time for the kids to go back to school. It was to be a new school for both of them. For Rebecca it was her first day of high school. It really was a significant time. Only a short time ago Leah doubted she would even see another Christmas and now many months on she was seeing her little girl grow up and start high school. We celebrated this wonderful time. The school was a wonderful environment for all of us. Leah was able to see Bim's first day at the Wilsons Creek school and Rebecca's first day of high school. Life had begun wonderfully in our new paradise. However, this was about to change, again. One evening, when I returned home from work, I found Leah on the floor in some distress. She looked like she had fainted but she hadn't. She had collapsed and didn't know what was happening. What was going on? I helped her up and she seemed to improve but I still needed to assist her and comfort her as she was in quite a panic. I then immediately got her to the doctors. We went to the quaint little hospital in Mullumbimby. It was only about ten minutes away. They kept Leah in for observation but couldn't come to any real conclusion. I was gutted. Leah was in obvious distress. I felt extremely guilty. Why had I left Leah? Why had I resumed work? These were crazy thoughts but, when faced with this guilt, they needed addressing. Was I selfish going back to work? I had to work, didn't I? We had bills to pay and life doesn't stand still just because someone had been sick in the past. I had actually applied for a carers benefit a while back to enable me to stay at home and help Leah stay healthy. But because Leah was so well I didn't qualify. Keeping Leah well wasn't reason enough for Leah to need help. Coming home and finding her on the floor made me realise that she did need help. We were in the middle of doing a renovation to create our beautiful little home. We were creating a safe place where Leah could focus on getting better in these magical surroundings. We would be able to finish what we were doing currently but the rest would have to wait for now. More pressing issues were ahead. Leah had been in great health recently. But with this new development I couldn't consider going back to work so I rang them to let them know what had happened. My employers were very understanding. The next day Leah was booked in for some tests and scans. The results weren't what we had wanted to hear. She had four new tumours. It was a sweet and sour moment. The good news is that her previous ones had gone as a result of the Gamma Knife. This treatment had done what nothing in Australia was capable of. This was a joyous moment in a funny sort of way. Over a year ago we had been given no options and Leah was told to get her affairs in order. The only possibility of help in Australia, whole head radiation, had only succeeded in diminishing Leah's health even further. It had no effect on her tumours in any way. But after one day of Gamma Knife treatment she had successfully had her tumours eradicated. Now to have four new ones emerge was so disappointing. Naturally we got on the phone to the Gamma Knife centre in the USA. We spoke to them and told them what had happened. They were perplexed. Apparently when the Gamma Knife is used to blast the tumours it renders that site in the brain incapable of having tumours grow back. These new ones were all in different places within the brain. They asked for us to immediately send the latest scans to San Diego to be assessed. We did this but it was bad news. The original tumours had in fact gone but four new tumours had sprouted up. The doctors were, as we were, quite disappointed. One tumour was actually quite large. This was now too big for the Gamma Knife to treat. Oh no, not again. We were gutted. We discussed options with Leah's oncologist. He basically shrugged his shoulders. Nothing had changed since we last asked for his help. There were still no options for us in Australia. Even four tumours in Australia were too many. Now Gamma Knife had been ruled out as well. Gamma Knife unfortunately does have its limitations. After numerous discussions, both here and overseas, it became clear that if the bigger tumour could be reduced in size Leah might have a better chance with Gamma Knife, but no guarantees. This gave us some hope. We discussed how we were to go about reducing the size of the biggest tumour with Leah's oncologist and a plan was devised which gave us some hope.

So we booked Leah in to a hospital in Melbourne for brain surgery. Again she was to travel away from home alone. At least she had family and friends in Melbourne. Leah was also again facing extremely invasive surgery with its associated risk. But it was quickly set up and she was ready to go quite soon after. She flew down and had the brain surgery but they couldn't get all of it due to its position in the brain, near the top of the spinal cord. Again this was surgery on the brain so it really knocked her about. She ended up being in Melbourne for a few weeks. She was depressed and weaker and the progress she had made over the past year or so seemed to be eradicated instantly. These were very frustrating times. Yet, again, Leah also amazed me. Every time a decision was made about Leah's health, be it mastectomy, brain surgery, chemo, radiation or Gamma Knife, she just took it in her stride. Even with the Gamma Knife she had actually had concerns about the cost. Now she was undergoing major brain surgery. She was brave and optimistic. There was no doubt about that. She was also a long way away. The children were back at school and I busied myself with tradesmen and renovations. This entire process in Melbourne took about six weeks. While all this was happening, I was trying to make sure the children continued relatively normal lives. We had begun the renovation on the home so it was quite chaotic in many aspects of our lives. Leah's health and wellbeing, of course, was of greatest concern. So I was juggling the renovation, which had now been scaled down, the kids lives and keeping up to date with what was happening to Leah many miles away. The operation was semi successful. But it was done. She spent some time in hospital and some time with her parents.

After Leah had recovered enough she returned to us. The portion of the renovation we decided to complete was practically finished so it was nice for her to be able to return to the lovely finished idea she had contributed so much to the design of. We still had a few finishing touches but it had been a total transformation. At least she missed out on the bedlam that had occurred during the renovation. We were living on a balcony for a while with only the BBQ to cook with and no lights. It was like a few weeks of camping. The children actually loved it and it took their minds of what was happening to mum. Soon Leah was home though. Our property was a bit hilly and Leah struggled somewhat to get around outside. This limited her to staying around the immediate house. She had lost some of the momentum she had gained directly after her Gamma Knife treatment. But she did have a big tumour that was creating pressure on her brain and spinal cord and no wonder she was a bit slower getting around. I was amazed she could even get out of bed in the mornings. Now we needed to get her well again. We had to get on to the Gamma Knife doctors, again, urgently. Leah contacted the Gamma Knife centre and they requested that she forward her new most recent scans. Thank goodness we now had these on disk and we could do all this via email. So Leah sent the scans and we waited in anticipation for the call so we could arrange the trip to San Diego for treatment. However we got bad news. They wouldn't be able to assist this time. The surgery had reduced the size of the biggest tumour but had made it impossible for the tumour to be treated with the Gamma Knife. I am still not sure of the exact reason for this but it had something to do with the surgery on the large tumour, location, and the effect the surgery had on Leah. This was a huge blow. Leah was inconsolable. I was amazed she had the energy to keep going. I was exhausted just watching. But she had the determination and the calmness to keep going. We contacted Leah's oncologist who again had to deliver the bad news. He had been optimistic that the Gamma Knife could help. If we had the Gamma Knife in Australia and she was able to keep close contact with the doctors using it, they may have picked up on the bigger tumour earlier, avoided surgery and maybe they could have treated the four new tumours. Who knows? But this was just a "what if" now. We were mortified. What had been such a positive year had just turned devastatingly bad. We had our beautiful life, Leah was enjoying it and now the future was cloudy again. Our saviours with the Gamma Knife couldn't help. Leah's oncologist couldn't help. Everyone we checked with couldn't help. I felt hopeless, helpless and drained. We felt extremely disadvantaged as we couldn't access this great technology, Gamma Knife, in Australia. We had the ability to make our way over to another country to access the treatment but didn't have access to the professionals using it in the meantime. Leah began to struggle with all this. She had been so strong. She had been able to cope with the emotional side of things as well as the physical. Now, however, the tumour was affecting her mobility. She would trip over occasionally. This would frustrate her immensely. The children were brilliant. They helped around the house and as we went to numerous appointments for various reasons they never complained. They would come along and sit patiently for hours if need be. The one positive thing was that the Gamma Knife had effectively killed many previous brain tumours so this gave us a glimmer of hope for the future. We just didn't know what or how at the time.

The bills began to mount as well. I was off work and Leah only had the disability benefit to rely on. I applied for a carers benefit again but still didn't qualify. Leah was too well to warrant requiring a carer. I was amazed. The next month was horrendous. Every avenue we went up turned into a dead end. Leah started to look to the future. A future without her in it. She was comforted, she told me, in the fact that if she were to go that the children would have me. I had done the role of mum and dad on many occasions and she felt comfortable that this would be fine for the future. It was quite emotional for all of us during that time. We had never been this low. This was also the first time we had confronted the future without Leah being a part of it. I hated this time of our lives. I now hated this journey which I would have quite happily not gone on. But again I needed to be strong and find a way. I don't consider myself an overly strong person. I am normally quite happy to just cruise along and go with the flow. But I drew on strength I didn't know I had for Leah and the children. We had started our new life and we needed to get through this and continue forward in this new paradise we had created. Now we needed another huge miracle. Was that greedy? Were we asking too much? I couldn't do this alone. I needed help. Leah needed this help as well. She was so strong and would endure anything but needed something to offer hope. At that moment she had very little.

# Chapter 17

# Cyberknife, dying to get to Oklahoma and even a tornado

Everything I investigated came back blank. This was such a frustrating time. Out of this frustration I decided to cast my net even wider. I stumbled upon a cancer support chat forum on the internet. I had asked every professional I could access, both in Australia and in the USA. Everyone had run out of options. The chat site had a diverse range of subjects and seemed a good source of information and support. I explained Leah's situation as best I could without actually posting her scans on the site. This felt like a long shot but one I had to take. I didn't even know if anyone would read my post. But in just a few hours I got a reply. It was suggested that we visit our local Cyberknife centre and ask their opinion. I should get the doctors at the Cyberknife centre to look at Leah's scans and offer their opinion. Cyberknife? I had never heard of it. I did a search. Not much information, in fact none in an Australian internet search. This was late at night so I couldn't really enquire elsewhere just yet. I did most of my research late at night as the rest of the day was busy with children, chores, appointments with Leah and such things. My head was clearer and I could concentrate more at night. The next day I made numerous phone calls about Cyberknife. Our doctor, both oncologists, one in Melbourne and one local and a number of hospitals. No one knew anything. I checked my spelling. I looked on the internet again to make sure this wasn't some kind of weird dream and Cyberknife was just invented during my sleep. Maybe I was barking up the wrong tree. I checked the spelling again, did some more Google searches and rang the doctors again. I could still not get any help. Then I got a private email. It was as a result of my cancer support chat. A doctor had replied via email as he didn't want to risk privacy issues by replying on the forum which was open to the public. Dr Medbery was a doctor using Cyberknife and he responded with a wealth of information on it. We had a look at the links he gave me on the internet. This was truly amazing stuff. Cyberknife was so advanced. It was sub millimetre accurate. A patient required no surgery. It's not really a knife it turns out. It uses a beam like a laser beam. Actually it uses hundreds of beams. Cyberknife is non invasive. A patient requires no drugs and there are no side effects. The patient is scanned and the scan fed in to a computer. This allows the robotic arm of the Cyberknife to administer beams to the exact site of the cancer from any of 360 degrees. Each beam goes in individually thus rendering them harmless but they meet up at the tumour and around 200 beams then do their job of destroying the cancer. The Cyberknife usually only takes one treatment session. The session only lasts about two or three hours. Cyberknife had similarities to Gamma Knife but no frame needed and it can treat the brain as well as lung, prostate, spine, liver and so many other tumours as well as cancer in children. We had a vague idea of its potential as Leah had already experienced the wonders of Gamma Knife. However we had no idea this technology existed. Until that day of course. Cyberknife used similar technology to Gamma Knife but was more recent, advanced and versatile. But again we didn't have it in Australia. It was 2006 and we were so far behind the rest of the world and people were being disadvantaged due to this fact. We asked a few more questions and then decided, if Leah was an acceptable candidate, to proceed. We were able to email Leah's scans to Dr Medbery as they were now on disk. He assessed them and it was decided they could treat all of Leah's tumours including the residual from her most recent brain surgery. It would actually take four days as the tumours would all need to be treated individually. Dr Medbery was almost apologetic for the treatment taking so long. Four days. Unbelievable. Other treatments take months and then months more to recover. We were reservedly ecstatic. It seemed a chance but we didn't want to get our hopes up too much. Leah was just so relieved to discover this option. It *was* a discovery. It was like we had discovered a planet such was the excitement and joy. But Leah sighed. She couldn't do all this again on her own. I had to be with her this time. It would be too much to expect another Jean Sweetwood to pop up in Oklahoma which is where we needed to go. Leah needed the support this time. There was no way I could say no.

We had enquired about the Cyberknife with what little information we could gather in Australia. Dr Medbery was a great help. Leah wanted him to perform the procedure. Dr Medbery was in Oklahoma City. We decided that would be the venue. We started preparations. It would take a bit to organise. It was a substantial cost, again, but what other alternatives were there? Maybe people with cancer should move permanently to another country while having treatment to get the best options and access. It was a bit late for us to contemplate this as a solution now. We would only go for the treatment which would be a short visit. We would have to fly to USA from Melbourne. We would take the children to Melbourne and pop them on a flight to Tasmania to stay with our great friends Anita and Byron, the children's God parents. The kids were excited. A holiday in Tasmania would be fun. They were obviously also apprehensive as they had seen this all too frequently in their short little lives so far. Then Leah and I would fly from Melbourne to Los Angeles. Connect to Colorado and then on to Oklahoma City. What a trek. We felt that it was amazing that a patient with brain tumours, quite a common illness in Australia, had to travel about thirty hours on a plane to the other side of the world for help. Now money was tight so we had to time it to perfection. With Cyberknife there is no need for hospital stays as it's such a gentle procedure but we had to stay somewhere. Cyberknife is actually a day procedure and most patients just have the treatment and go home. I checked on the internet and found a semi self contained hotel suite with complimentary breakfast not far from the hospital. I booked that for ten nights which seemed to be the length of stay we would need, so the doctors said.

We were set. We felt like pioneers. Off, again, into the great unknown.

Our local media had heard about Leah's plight. Alex from the Lismore newspaper arranged for a story to be done. He came out with a photographer and composed a story about us and the entire family had a photo taken to accompany the story. We thought this might be another round of publicity highlighting the lack of options available in Australia. What amazed Alex was the prevalence of these treatments in other countries around the world. Cyberknife was in 200 hospitals worldwide at that time. Places like India had several hospitals offering Cyberknife. Japan had about 20 hospitals offering it. We had no idea the impact this publicity would bring. After the visit from the journalist we got ready to go. We were all set. We packed our bags. That in itself was a big task. We had to pack for the whole family heading off to different destinations. Once packed, we headed to Gold Coast airport for our initial flights to Melbourne. We were so nervous. I was a bundle of nerves. I can only imagine how terrified Leah was.

At Melbourne airport the children would then board as unaccompanied minors onto their connecting flight to Hobart. We had to wait with them until they boarded. Saying goodbye to them was one of the hardest things I had done in my life. I had only been away from them once before for such a long period. I don't know how Leah had done it so often. But she wanted to see them grow up so the sacrifice was worth it in her mind. After the children were in the air we then transferred to the International terminal for our big trip ahead. At this stage of our lives we had little money at our disposal but as we had both been working for most of the previous year we were able to pop the flights for all of us on our credit cards. We were prime candidates for the banks. A married couple, working with low debt at the time, so money to pay for Leah's treatments was easy to access. We would worry about repaying it when we returned and Leah was better. Money was the least of our worries at that moment. This same thought had crossed our minds before but we had managed. Leah felt a bit guilty about all this expense but I told her not to worry. Our only concern was to get her better. I felt let down by the fact we didn't have these treatments in Australia. Someone with cancer shouldn't feel guilty about accessing treatment. It was just a shame the treatment was so far away. We were also lucky that Leah was in relatively good shape and was able to travel such a distance. She had struggled with the flight from Melbourne to Hamilton Island after her radiation treatment but had no such experience coming back from San Diego after Gamma Knife. The doctors in Oklahoma had suggested the same ease of travel should be expected after Cyberknife. We were amazed.

I didn't know much about Oklahoma. I researched a bit to see what we could expect. It was nice to be researching something nice for a change. It made a difference to all the cancer research I had done over the years. Oklahoma looked quite interesting. They had the Cowboy Museum which had a lot of information about people like Ronald Reagan, the former US President. The airport is the Roy Rogers airport. The city was the scene of the tragic Oklahoma bombing. Leah had given me a book a few years previously. It was called "1001 things to do before you die". I still laugh at the title. This was a travel book covering the highlights of destinations around the world. We had done numerous of these. We'd had a Las Vegas wedding, been to the beautiful Santorini in the Greek Isles. We had visited Disneyland and had even lived near the Great Barrier Reef in Australia. We looked to see what Oklahoma had to offer. A world famous steak restaurant was all that was in the book for Oklahoma. Well if that was it for Oklahoma, we would do it.

It took nearly 30 hours of travelling to get to Oklahoma City. There was the 4 hour wait for connections in Los Angeles to get to Colorado and another few hours at Colorado before our flight to Roy Rogers airport. We got there and got a shuttle to our hotel. We didn't even stop for food as we were both exhausted. We had some big days coming up. We asked the shuttle driver to pick us up in the morning, he would become our driver. It was a bit more expensive but at least we knew he'd be there for us each day and we couldn't afford to miss a session as we were on a tight schedule. The hospital was about 20 minutes away. There wasn't much traffic in the suburbs of Oklahoma City, so negotiating it was easy. We slept for hours once we arrived at our hotel. When we woke, on that first morning, we were starving and breakfast was included so we strolled down to the breakfast room prior to our trip to the hospital. It was a true American breakfast. We ate off paper plates. There were thermos flasks of coffee. We drank out of disposable cups, used stirrers and added coffee whitener. The accompanying juice was reconstituted. But the food was alright. They offered eggs, bacon, cereal, toast, pancakes and waffles. It hit the spot and before we knew it our driver was there to take us to meet the experts who would guide us through the Cyberknife treatment. This first day was just a planning and information session. They would explain to us the procedure and answer any questions we had. We were both nervous. This was like an opening night of a play or an audition. We had brought some Australian wine and stuffed koalas for the staff. The doctor had been to Australia and visited the Barrier reef near where we used to live so we felt some good Aussie souvenirs were appropriate as an early thank you. We walked in to the hospital and we were immediately amazed. It was like a shopping mall. It didn't resemble a hospital at all. It had lush waiting rooms with coffee and biscuits. The suites were amazing. The floors were covered with lovely carpet. We were able to read current edition magazines. There was cable television in most rooms. The entire hospital had warm lighting and an almost inviting atmosphere. The only thing that reminded us that we were in a hospital was the uniforms of the staff. We met all the staff who would be involved. The main two were Dr Medbery and his assistant Deborah. They were just so wonderful, informative and compassionate. We felt at ease with them straight away. Leah felt confident immediately. They showed us the facility and set up the week's events. It was actually quite a relief to have these two looking after Leah. As this technology was so foreign to us they took time to show us all the components, the staff involved and to explain the process. The next day Leah would have the first of her scans. We both felt extremely comfortable now seeing this state of the art facility and the professional staff that would be delivering the treatment. Leah began to cry but they were tears of joy. A few weeks earlier she was facing death for a second time and now she had a solution. We now had to go to the finance department to pay for the scans. This was the hardest part. The actual treatment was going to be easy. After forking over the money for the numerous scans requested we had the rest of the day free. We said our goodbyes and headed off to the buzz of Oklahoma City. We did a little bit of grocery shopping so we could have some snacks in our room. We visited a

Walmart which I had never been to before. It was absolutely amazing. Not necessarily in a good way. It offered a huge choice and how any small retailers could survive with such a cheap one stop shop is beyond me. Healthy options weren't high on their list of priorities but we were able to get some fruit and yoghurt. We even bought a proper cup for our morning tea or coffee. We were already over the paper cups, on offer at most places we visited, in which they served the coffee. There were lots of things to get used to in this part of the world. I was beginning to get an understanding of how alone and scared Leah must have been when she went to San Diego and, again, how grateful I was that she had Jean to help her on that trip. Things overseas are quite different and to have to deal with all that and a cancer treatment must have taken a special person. Leah was that person. I was proud to be assisting her at this time. She did need a bit of assistance. The pressure on the brain had made walking for Leah quite difficult. In a straight line she was fine even if a bit slow. But any kerbs, steps or obstacles and she risked tripping and falling. I was there to help. We must have looked like an old pensioner couple. We were in no great hurry though so the shuffle served its purpose.

Oklahoma City is about the size of Brisbane in Australia. It is more spread out. Downtown is really just the business district. It doesn't offer a great deal to entice you. The suburbs are where most of the action is. The suburbs have the restaurants, shopping malls, parks and facilities. The route to the airport is where many of the tourist activities are. It has the tourist hotels, restaurants and more shopping. The area where we were staying had a shopping centre, all the take away chains, a Walmart and not much else. It was so different to any part of the USA we had seen before. It was on Route 66.

It had a real country or rural feel about it yet they had three hospitals offering Cyberknife, many Gamma Knife centres as well and other treatments we don't have in Australia. Doctors and oncologists actually have an arsenal of solutions for people with cancer in even the smallest of cities in America. However I found it hard to find a decent cup of coffee and that was one thing we do better in Australia. We may have great coffee but better cancer care options would be a more desirable situation I am thinking. We had found great cancer care, I'm sure we would find a decent cup of coffee. We gave up on the coffee for the moment and we went back to our hotel and rested as the next day was going to be a big day.

We discovered that I was right. The next day was a huge day for Leah. We got up, took our real mugs down to the breakfast room, had breakfast and got our shuttle to the hospital. This was day one of the process which would rid Leah of this cancer. Leah had gone backwards since her surgery in Melbourne a few weeks ago. She had lost a bit of mobility. Stepping up a gutter or stair was sometimes difficult. She tripped a few times with all the moving around we were doing. She was happy and motivated but she got a bit frustrated with her physical restrictions. She had achieved so much after her Gamma Knife treatment but felt as if she was back at square one. The tumours were causing this but the Cyberknife would rectify it. At the hospital it was time for Leah's scans. They were done on another floor to where the Cyberknife was. We had to go to a different department and wait for Leah's turn. Just as in Australia, there was still a lot of sitting around and waiting. We got to read many magazines and the local newspapers. We got to meet the locals. We were able to have some brilliant chats. But eventually the scans were done and Leah was one step closer to her first Cyberknife treatment. The scans were transferred to the Cyberknife department and we went and had lunch in the hospital cafeteria while we waited for the next step. The cafetreia was more like a food court. It had such an amazing choice. And the gift shop had espresso coffee. We had made another great discovery. It was also a great place to meet more people. Some were also in for Cyberknife. We shared stories. Everyone laughed at us because we had to come all the way from Australia to li'l ole Oklahoma for treatment. Some of the people we met had never even travelled outside of Oklahoma. Some had not seen the ocean as Oklahoma is slap bang in the middle of the USA. We were amazed by these trinkets of knowledge and they were amazed by our journey. It was quite funny at the time. It was also nice to see Leah laughing. We chatted to a man who had a tumour behind his eye. He was having Cyberknife which was administered straight through the eye without any anesthetic. Each beam went through the eye individually and then they all met up at the tumour. This is where the Cyberknife did its work. No pain. No discomfort. No side effects. We were amazed.

I met another lady who went through what Leah was going through at that moment. This lady went in to receive her Cyberknife treatment. She was all set up, she was on the treatment table, time went by and she asked "when are you going to commence the treatment?" The doctors informed her that they'd finished. Well we all rolled around laughing. I was so happy for Leah to hear these stories as any anxiety just slipped away. Next, though, it was time for Leah to meet the doctors. We returned from lunch for the treatment plan. As Leah had four tumours she would get a scan for one tumour and have treatment the next day. This would be the procedure for all four tumours. So they had the scans for the first tumour and Leah would have her first Cyberknife treatment the next morning. She had a mixture of nervousness and excitement. We left the hospital again and returned to the hotel in anticipation of what the next new day would bring. I will deviate just for a second here.

While waiting for Leah's first meeting with the Cyberknife we were watching some local television. One show caught my eye. It was a medical program. Two doctors were chatting about why we are still quite large even after eradicating fat and sugar from our diets. They went on to mention how everything is fat free and sugar free yet we still have increased cases of cancer, diabetes as well as other diseases. They said that with eliminating fat and sugar from foods something had to be added to give it flavor. The one constant that made sense of all their research was modified corn. Corn meal, corn starch, corn syrup, corn chips and many other items were examples of modified corn. Americans consume huge amounts of these products. Just about everything you pick up at the supermarket has some form of modified corn in it. They consume litres of diet drinks with no sugar but they all have corn syrup in its place. This was an interesting thought. Something I take with me when I do the grocery shopping. I must stress that they did mention that fresh corn is okay as its not modified. But this was a definite eye opener which we stumbled upon by chance. Now I will continue with our adventure with Cyberknife.

We returned in the morning and sat in the waiting room. The staff came and escorted Leah to the room where the Cyberknife would do its stuff. I was allowed to go with her until the actual treatment would begin. I was lucky to be able to meet the machine that was going to rid my wife of her cancer. I was also able to comfort Leah while she waited for the treatment to commence. They got Leah to lie down on a body shaped, treatment table. It had a small square base under her head. They stretched a netted material over her face and head and attached it to the square base on the bed. This was to hold her head still while the treatment was in progress. It's how they would get the accuracy. They asked Leah what music she would like to listen to. She requested Dean Martin. I was so proud of her. We loved Deano. It also made the entire process very individual for Leah. We felt this differed to treatment in Australia which is almost mass produced. Then, when it was all ready, I was asked to leave the room. The staff double checked everything and they also left and then we gathered around the monitor in the control room. It was basically a screen, a computer and the controls. This was where they controlled the treatment, monitored its progress, observed and communicated with Leah. I could watch it on the screen. It was amazing to watch the robotic arm moving around any of the 360 degrees to ensure the best access to kill this first tumour. Before we knew it the treatment was over. It took just over two hours. They took the netting off Leah's head. They allowed her to rest and then she was sent on her way. She had no discomfort. She had no effects. The worst thing that happened was that she had little indentations on her skin from the netting that had held her head in place. This disappeared in about 15 minutes. Leah had found it less claustrophobic than the Gamma Knife as she was actually positioned inside chamber with the Gamma Knife. With the Cyberknife she was out in the open and she found it quite relaxing. We then went shopping. We left, to return the next day for a new scan prior to Leah's second treatment. This all seemed so simple.

We went in the next day and all hell had broken loose. The hospital had been inundated by the media wanting to do a story on Leah. They were amazed by two things. One was that Australia didn't have advanced treatments such as this and the other was that we had come all the way to Oklahoma to make use of the treatment. Leah went for her scan and the representatives from the media arranged a suitable time to interview her. It was decided that Leah would have a few more treatments first as even after the first one she seemed to be a lot better physically. The better she was, the better the interview would be for all concerned. So at this stage she had her second scan and then the next day her second tumour was treated with the Cyberknife. After this treatment Leah wanted a change of scenery so we went out to the tourist area for a lunch at the Hard Rock Cafe. Amazing. After a cancer treatment her vitality was such that she wanted to see a bit of Oklahoma. I also noted how much better her mobility was after just the second treatment. This was amazing. We also went shopping and bought things for the children as gifts for when we returned. Even though the exchange rate was low for our Australian dollar at the time, making everything including the costs at the hospital almost double, basic things here were so cheap. So that day we shopped, ate and then returned home to the hotel to rest. The next day brought more of the same. Another scan and then we did some sightseeing. This time we visited the memorial to the Oklahoma bombing. This was so emotional. So many people, including many children were killed. The memorial was very well done with a place of reflection, plaques dedicated to the victims and amazing information about the event. I had heard a bit of it in Australia but this made it more personal. It was very moving. Oklahoma was quite a discovery. It was a big country town with a city feel and an unusual history. The Oklahoma bombing was now an unfortunate part of that history. Oklahoma was now part of our history. The following day Leah had her next Cyberknife treatment and then we fronted the media. ABC TV news filmed us with Dr Medbery and the daily Oklahoma newspaper wrote a story as well. We were more than happy to oblige. If we could use this when we got home to help the cause to bring Cyberknife to Australia, all the better. We were adamant that we would campaign for Cyberknife to be brought to Australia as we were truly amazed. The effect, or lack of, was noticeable. Leah was more alert, moving freely and her appetite was back. While Leah was having her scans or treatment I would wait in the waiting room. I would chat with people about their stories after they had ascertained ours. I met one lady who had been bed ridden with spinal tumours before Cyberknife came to Oklahoma. Now she walked in for her treatments and maintained a normal lifestyle, except for her yearly visits for a "clean up". She stressed that she was not cured but as the effects of Cyberknife were few she was able to have continual treatments to maintain a good quality of life. I laughed that other treatments weren't really cures either but the side effects made for poor quality of life. She agreed. How lucky was this lady? That was the thought that went through my mind at the time. I saw her as lucky yet she had cancer! This was how messed up my thoughts had become during this journey with Leah. Of course the lady with spinal tumours wasn't lucky. But she was able to access this great treatment and have follow up visits with the specialists at her leisure. If Cyberknife was available in Australia Leah may have had the same opportunity. We could have had numerous sessions for the same price as the trip to Oklahoma. She may have avoided the destructive whole brain radiation that nearly killed her and used up nine months of Leah's life with no result. I was beginning to get quite frustrated with what was on offer back home. Not just for Leah but for everyone. I heard stories of children being treated with Cyberknife without pain, drugs, side effects or surgery.

I had visited chemotherapy wards in Australia and sometimes I couldn't stay. The wards had a morose atmosphere at the best of times. This hospital was different. We sat around drinking coffee, laughing, sharing stories and remaining so optimistic. Even the staff members were extremely upbeat. The staff in Australia were amazing as well and I'm sure, if they had Cyberknife to work with, they would be even more successful. I had noted, in the past though, the frustration of some hospital staff at the hopelessness of some cases but they never flinched in their desire to provide the best they could for all patients. They deserved technology like Cyberknife as much as the patients and families did. After each session with the Cyberknife I noticed a marked improvement in the little things with Leah's health. She was already walking so much better. We spent a full day at the mall after one session. We had lunch at the Cattleman's restaurant which was the big steakhouse in the book "1001 things to do before you die". We had to queue up to get in and it was only 11.30am. Leah ordered a huge steak and since she had been basically vegetarian for a number of years this was a big surprise on two fronts:

- She usually ate like a rabbit due to the effects of treatments and her tiredness and that is why I tried to make each meal as high in nutrient and protein as possible.

- The enthusiasm in which she ordered and then devoured this steak was something I hadn't seen in ages. It may have been the only thing featured in Oklahoma, in the book, but it was definitely one of the most memorable.

After another Cyberknife session we visited the cowboy museum. Leah was so much more vital in just a few short days. A number of hours looking at the history of the relationship between the local Indian population and the cowboys, who were famous from this area, was rewarding and extremely fascinating. It was amazing that the former US president Ronald Reagan featured so prominently here. A local man heard our voices and asked where we were from and we said Australia and he responded with. Auf Wiedersehen. It wasn't until weeks later I worked out he thought we were from Austria not Australia. We both laughed at this with fondness when we had returned to Australia. The museum had a lovely cafe so we rested and had a nice afternoon tea there which topped off a memorable experience. This was cancer treatment as I'd never witnessed before.

With the number of scans Leah needed, as well as the treatments, we were fearful that we may have to re schedule our return flights. We had scheduled things quite tightly due to the cost of everything. We needed accommodation, meals and transfers and these cost quite a bit each day. So we had worked out with the staff, prior to coming over, how long we would need to stay. But now, with the weekend coming up, we were running out of time. Then to our amazement the hospital said they would keep the Cyberknife centre open on the weekend to prevent us having to change plans. Everything was falling in to place. We were amazed by these wonderful people and the technology. It was well worth our trip to the other side of the world. We were almost done with Leah's treatment and then we would be free to return home to Australia. It was all quite simple really. Maybe things were going too well? We returned, after a visit to the hospital, to our hotel and we were just relaxing in our room and having a snack and a cuppa. We had the television on and a major commotion broke out. The program on the television disappeared and sirens began wailing. We were shocked at first but soon discovered it was a tornado warning siren. It was getting dark and gloomy outside. I rang reception and asked what we should do but he had no idea. He was a great help in a totally foreign situation for us. We had come all around the world for Leah to get better and we were about to get snuffed out by a tornado? Great. I had a quick peek out the front door. It was extremely windy. But the apartment building next door seemed very calm. People having cigarettes on balconies paying no heed to the commotion happening around them. I remember hearing stories of cyclone Tracey in Darwin in Australia many years ago and the survivors said to stay away from windows and to move under a support such as a door way. The bathroom in our room was the best place. We went in and sat on the floor and as it had no window at all in there we felt safe for the moment. The siren on the television and also outside continued for about 45 minutes. It was a time that we could reflect on the past. We laughed about how surreal all this felt at present and we pondered the future. It passed the time as this natural menace wove it's magic outside. Then we heard voices. It was the newsreader on the television. The sirens had stopped. We ventured out of our safe haven and took a look outside. Not much carnage here, lots of rubbish and some light items outside had been disturbed a bit but not too bad. However on the news it was a different story. Aeroplanes at the airport had been tipped over, roofs ripped off houses, boats on lakes damaged. I think we had been on the far perimeter of the tornado and people in the direct route of it were hardest hit. It amazed me that we had to endure this scary situation just so Leah could get cancer treatment that we should have in Australia anyway. Most people just have to worry about getting a car park prior to receiving their cancer treatment but Leah had to dodge a tornado. It was in the newspapers the next day so I bought a copy to bring home. Oh, there was a story on Leah and I in there as well!!!

Leah's treatment was soon over. Cyberknife can treat a patient in as little as a few hours. She required the four treatments due to having four tumours but she suffered no ill effects and actually improved in the short time we were in Oklahoma. She was given a final look over and given the okay to travel. The farewell was quite emotional. The staff had all become like family. But Leah's treatment was over. It was time to go home. So we braced ourselves for the huge journey home. But at the end of that long trip would be our children. Oklahoma had provided us with a lifetime of experiences and the challenge of bringing Cyberknife to the notice of the people that could instigate change back in Australia. Leah was so frustrated that she had gone through a number of invasive procedures and some that had been ineffective. She may not have needed to do all of that if Cyberknife was available in Australia. This would have resulted in less impact on her body over the last few years. If available in Australia Leah would not have needed to be away from her family so often and for so long. Our family would not have been subjected to the expense associated with receiving these treatments overseas. She now realised that she may not benefit from getting Cyberknife to Australia as she had already endured the trip to Oklahoma to receive it. Leah, however, wanted to make sure other Aussies who couldn't raise the money or were unable to travel could access this at home. I agreed.

# Chapter 18

# Home again, what could go wrong?

It may have taken a while but we were finally home. The children were so glad to see us and the feeling was mutual. We had rung the children every day, once we worked out the time difference, while we were away. Byron and Anita were amazing and made sure it was like a real holiday while the children were in Tasmania. The kids even helped Anita give up smoking by hiding her cigarettes.

We were back in our new home. The children were settled in at their new schools. Life could hopefully become normal again. I still wasn't working so I could help Leah return to her normal self. This was already beginning to happen. Leah was also very keen to get the word out about Cyberknife. The day we returned I got a phone call from a mother whose eight year old son had a brain tumour. She had seen our story in the local paper which was available online so even though she was in Brisbane she had heard about our journey to find Cyberknife. I explained it all to her and she was excited. However they had already operated on her son. The operation had created the need for a plate to be inserted in his skull. This plate had made international travel impossible due to the pressurised atmosphere in the planes. It was totally frustrating because if we had it in Australia she would still be able to access Cyberknife, even if it meant driving to another city to get it. An international flight was out of the question for this family. It wasn't fair. This became a common theme. We got numerous enquiries. We were contacted by people who may have been in similar situations, others from people who had lost loved ones and wanted to help. One man had just lost his wife. She had basically died from the radiation treatment she had been subjected to. The husband was disgusted with what she had to endure when less invasive treatments were available overseas. His two children, in their 20's, have a genetic possibility to also get their mums cancer. So this man wanted to assist in getting Cyberknife to Australia so his children had more options for the future if needed. We sent letters out. We spoke with media contacts we knew. I wrote letters to the newspapers but not much changed. In the meantime we had Leah to nurture back to her old self. She continued her meditation, dietary regime, maintained her nutrients and the well developed rituals she took part in. We walked and we both benefitted from that. Life was good. We lived in a lovely valley, in a lovely house with lovely friends and neighbours. This was what it was all about. Our local media heard of Leah's quest to get this treatment to Australia. They were aware of her need to go to Oklahoma from the story written before we went. They came to do a follow up story. Leah explained it all from her point of view. The journalist was amazed. Leah had undergone brain treatment only a few days ago, then travelled thirty hours to get home, but seemed fine. We said we needed to get this treatment to Australia. The journalist said we needed a Cyberknife in every capital city. If only the rest of the country thought the same.

Leah was progressing well. We saw the kids doing well at school. We had a lovely Easter with family who flew up from Melbourne. I was looking for work again due to how well Leah was going. Months had passed now since the trip to Oklahoma. Leah and I had been to the beach for a walk on the sand. It had been good to strengthen her muscles. She was quite fit at that moment. We were both getting lots of fresh air and exercise. I think even I was getting fitter. It may not have been the beach each day as we were spoilt for choice. We could walk a country road or through the rainforest. When we got home we would make some fresh juice, some of the fruit and vegetables we were now growing. The produce in our local stores was of amazing quality anyway. We visited the many farmers markets that the region had to offer. We could get wholefoods in bulk locally as well which was a cheaper option. Leah would retire to our expansive deck, with views over the rainforest to the ocean, to meditate or do some yoga. Leah painted and did mosaics. She found these activities very therapeutic. Friends came over and took part as well. It was a great period in both of our lives. But this day we had been to the beach. On the way home we needed to stop at the medical centre in town to get a prescription so Leah could get that filled at the chemist. We went in to the medical centre and waited. When it was her turn Leah got up and went in. As she sat down she got light headed. She fainted and they had trouble waking her. She was groggy. I was freaking out, anxious and scared. They called an ambulance and had her transferred to Lismore hospital which was about 45 minutes away. I had to go home and get the children and then we met Leah at the hospital. When we got there Leah was in the emergency room but sitting up and hooked up to a few monitors. She seemed alright. She was frightened. It was another new situation. Leah could cope with the stuff she new and had previously experienced but this was a new and unexpected situation. They were doing a few tests. We waited to see what was happening. The doctors said for us to go home as the results could be some time. Leah seemed fine so we did go and I would come back the next day. Nothing appeared too serious so at this stage I didn't call anyone. It was a matter of waiting. However, when I returned the next day she was worse. She had been moved to a ward. Apparently her liver had failed. I went to the ward to see her. She was tired but could still chat and knew what was happening. I stayed with her a while then left for home to meet the children. I explained that mum was still at the hospital. I rang Leah's parents and explained what had happened. They booked to come up from Melbourne. I took the children in to the hospital but Leah was very tired so we didn't stay too long. Leah's parents flew in to Ballina about 45 minutes away from Lismore. I met them and we returned to the hospital. They were stunned. They hadn't seen Leah like this. We spoke with doctors and they explained about the liver failure. They were trying what they could to help her but didn't hold out much hope. What was going on? Leah had beaten every obstacle thrown at her. Now she had another setback to deal with. We spoke to doctors about options. They were medicating her and monitoring her but little response. It was a wait and see situation. Leah's parents stayed with us. We would travel in each morning on the 45 minute drive to Lismore. I had taken the children out of school so they could be around Leah and give her hugs and support. We would stay all day and chat. We would help feed her, hold hands and help Leah in any way we could. Things didn't improve though.

A dear friend from Rosebank, Jacinta who I have spoken about earlier, took time out to come and look after the children as it was all a bit much and boring for them. She would take them to the park and her assistance was invaluable. She would sit with us and pray that Leah would get better.

We waited and waited for improvement but it wasn't coming. The liver was really struggling and this was putting a strain on other parts of the body. I had found solutions in the past so used my down time to try and do the same now. We would all leave the hospital at around 7pm, head home and have some dinner in silence. We were a devastated family. This was actually the first time we had all dealt with it while living together. It was another twist in this journey. My aunt and uncle dropped in while on their journey home from Queensland to Melbourne after visiting their daughter and her family. They stayed and offered support and comfort. It was so nice of them. It was a time that people helped any way they could from wherever they were. The nights were the worst. We were stunned. After everyone was in bed I would research options. A transplant of the liver was out of the question. People who have had cancer, and this was secondary cancer for Leah, were not candidates due to the shortage of donor livers which are saved for otherwise healthy patients. An artificial liver is available but it is really only for people awaiting transplants whose liver has shut down and this arrangement acts as the liver for a short time until a new liver can be found. Stem cells were looked at. An Australian group had done research into stem cells in reproducing the liver. I rang about this but as this was done by Australians in conjunction with a German group all the information was in Germany. We looked at a care flight to get Leah to a major city such as Sydney or Brisbane but she was considered not well enough to travel. All the medical options I could find returned negative. I decided to go down a different path. I rang some of Leah's childhood friends and three of them flew up for the weekend. They were obviously devastated to see Leah like this. They said they would help in any way they could. They shared funny stories and cried and laughed. Leah was quite alert during this stay which was wonderful. I think the visit had stimulated Leah quite significantly. We shared a gin and tonic. Our entire family was comforted by these wonderful girls who had come so far to be with their sick friend. It was a bitter sweet time. They stayed for the weekend. Leah was asleep for some of it, awake at other times but buoyed by their presence. It was good to see the improvement in Leah. However this couldn't last forever. The girls had to return home. The girls left and then it was week two of Leah's stay in hospital.

What would be the solution? No one had any answers or solutions. I have never felt so helpless in all my life. Leah had been in hospital about ten days, she had gotten much weaker and interacted only occasionally and then she gently passed away. That was it. We had run out of options and Leah had run out of fight. This was the saddest day indeed. I just broke down. The staff involved in caring for Leah broke down. Everyone broke down. We had remained strong for so long but Leah's passing created a wave of devastation. Leah had fought a battle I would have only had the strength to battle part of. She had left everyone in awe of her spirit, attitude and pluck. But she was not scared of the next place and enough was enough. It was July 2006. Leah had been sliced up, burnt by radiation, poisoned, prodded and probed. Her body had been battered and bruised for too long but she was still beautiful. All the invasive treatments Leah had endured couldn't take her beauty away. Her body may have been broken but the wonderful woman would remain in our hearts and memories. At least she was at peace now and had to battle no more. We did reflect on how, like people such as Elvis and Marilyn Monroe, Leah would be remembered as young - never to grow old.

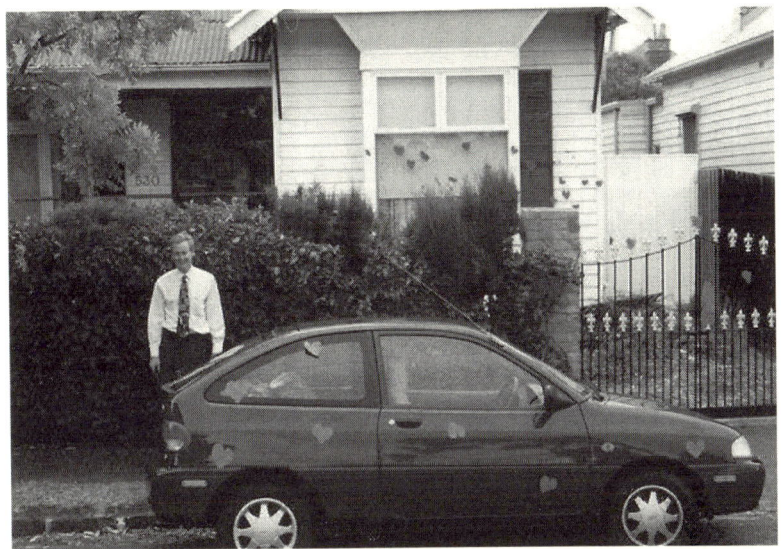

Valentines Day - When it all began

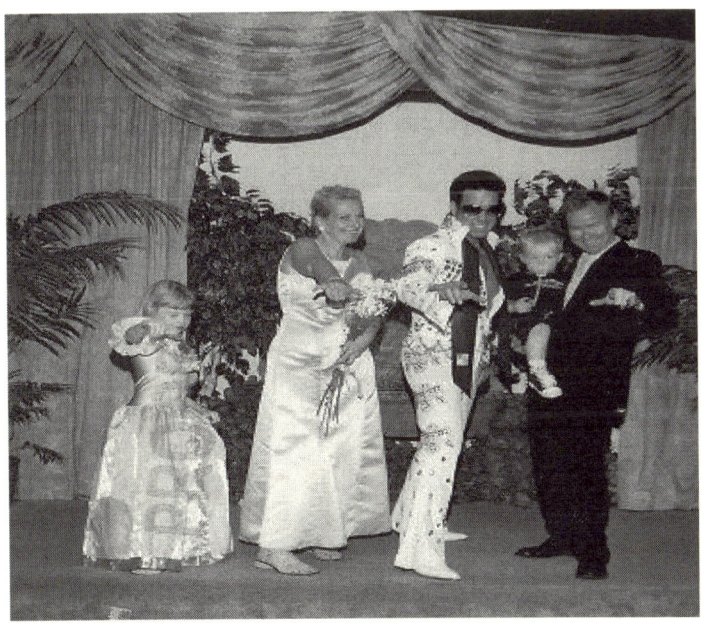

Our wedding day in Vegas with Elvis. It was great to have the kids involved

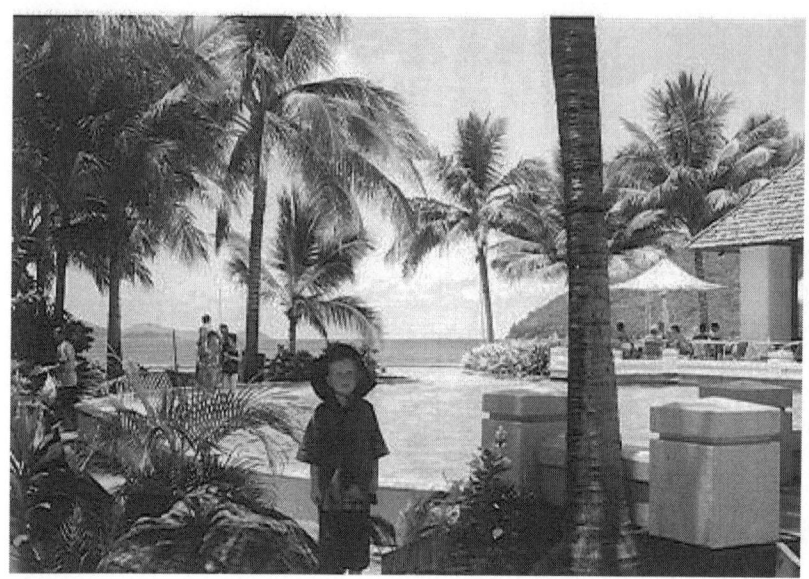

Bim's first day of school on Hamilton Island

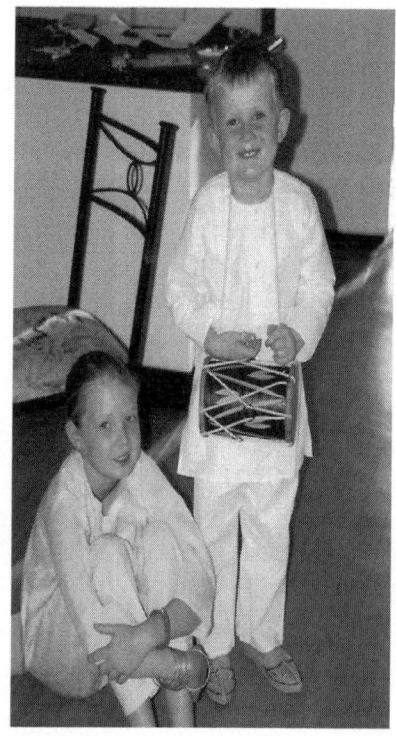

The kids fitted out after our trip to India

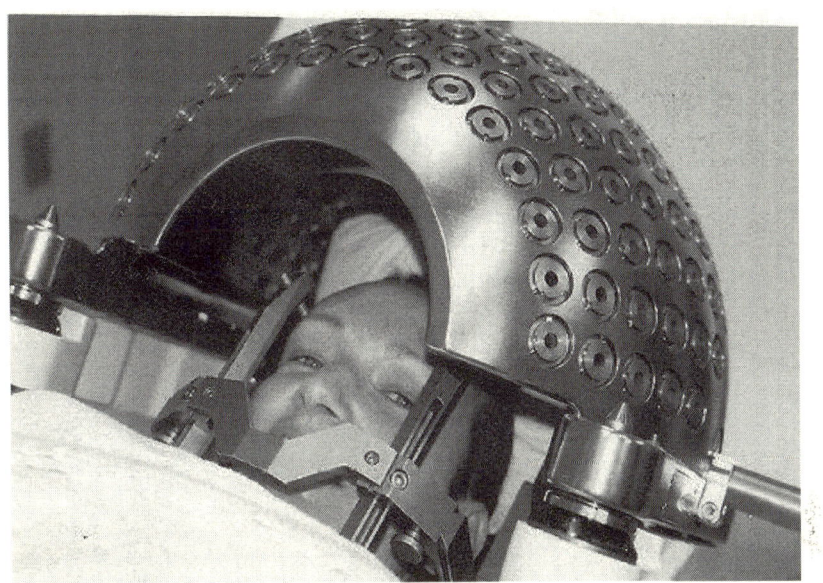

Leah ready for the Gamma Knife

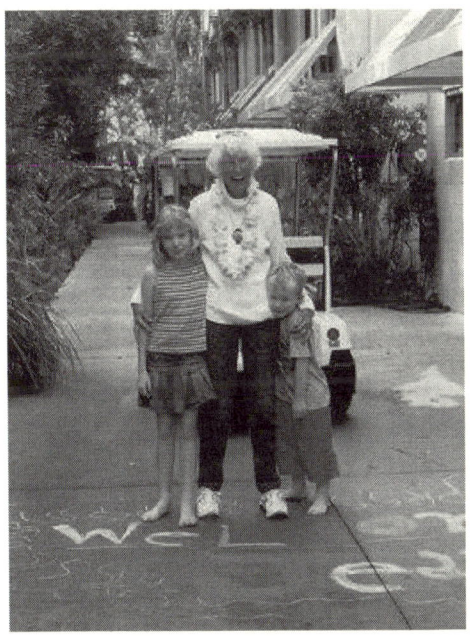

We all welcomed Jean to our home on Hamilton Island

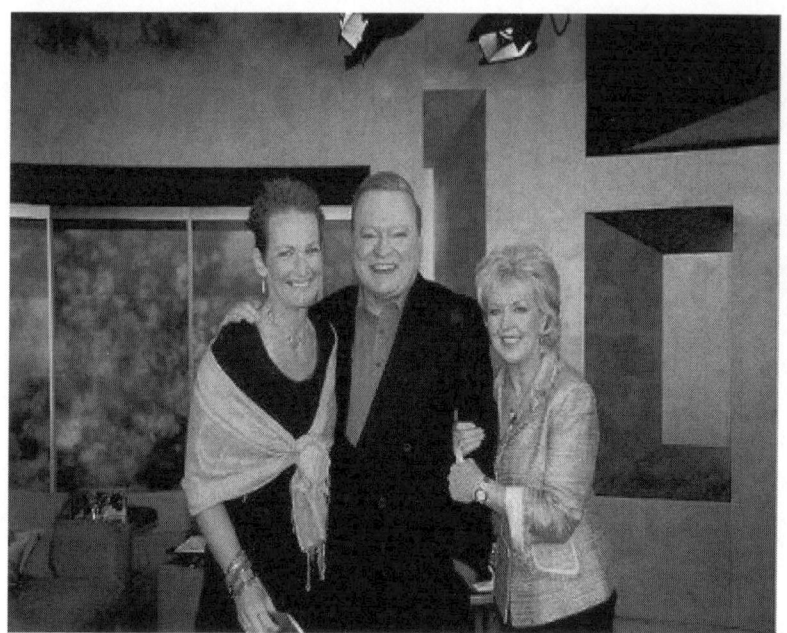

Leah on the set of Good Morning Australia with Bert and Patti

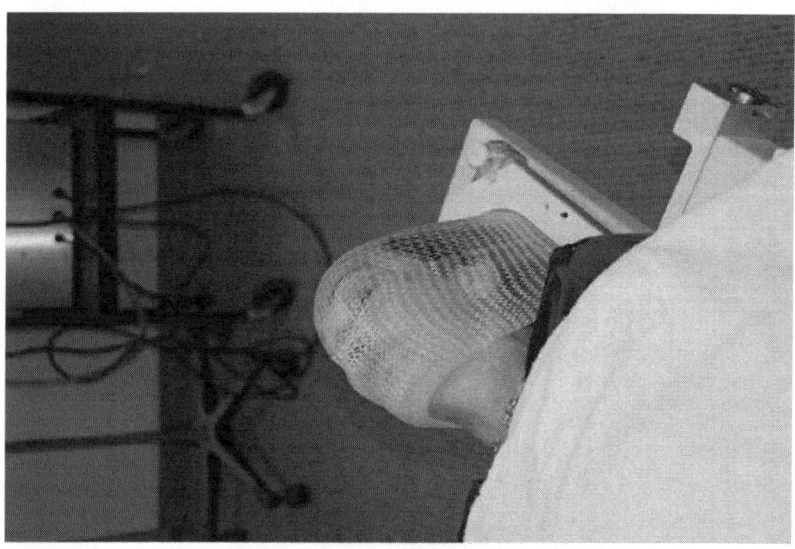

Leah prepared for the Cyberknife

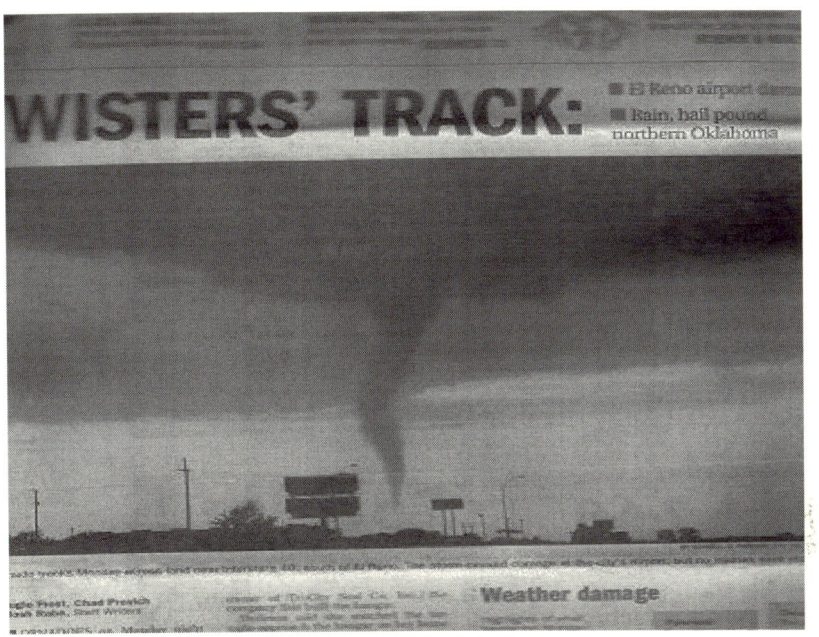

The tornado in the news the day after we lived through it

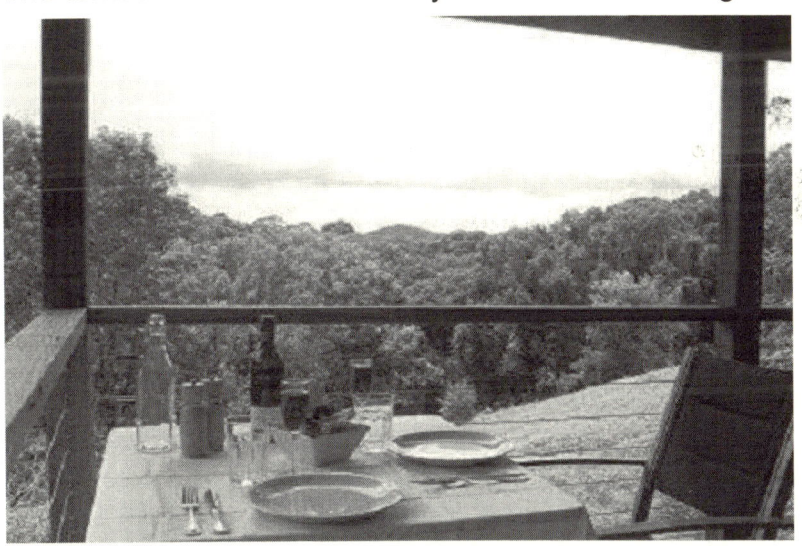

Leahbelles via Byron Bay. Could have been yours for $100

# Chapter 19

# What next?

Dr Seuss once said **"don't be sad that it's over, be happy that it happened".** I wished I could have lived those words in the days after Leah's death. However I was now overwhelmingly numb. I was totally out of puff. Shattered. I think I went into melt down. We had faced cancer full on and succeeded each time, even when we were told nothing could be done. Leah had been so brave. But it had all ended. It was like the battle was all for nothing. I didn't know what to do. I was lost. I had no energy and very little enthusiasm. But you don't get time to dwell or be still. We had to have a funeral for Leah. However I couldn't do anything to help. Nothing. The funeral was organised, by Leah's parents, to be in a chapel in Melbourne. It was just down the road from the hotel where Leah and I had first met. This was going to be so hard. We would hold a gathering at the hotel after the service. We wanted and needed a chance to catch up with friends and family spread all over the country. Leah deserved a celebration as well. She needed to have the send off she had the right to.

People needed the opportunity to pay their respects. The children were so scared. They didn't understand. We had gone through so much that you'd think we would have been ready for this day. But nothing prepares you for it. I had been in a daze since Leah's death. Leah's parents had returned to Melbourne to arrange the funeral. We were left alone. My role had now changed. The children were frightened to think that we would have to move. They had just lost their mum and now they feared they'd lose their home and their friends to. I assured them that this would not be the case. I didn't know how but I would have to manage. I didn't even have the energy to think of such things at the moment. But we needed to get organised to get to Leah's funeral.

Earlier in the year Leah and I had booked flights to Melbourne for September to visit friends and family. We had done this without even thinking anything would prevent the trip as she had been improving so well. We thought we would pay a visit to friends and family down there together as she had travelled solo the last few times due to her treatment needs. After her death I approached Jetstar, the airline the tickets were booked with, to change Leah's ticket to Rebecca so she could go to her mum's funeral. They refused to budge. It was the cheap fare that we had paid and these were non transferable. I pleaded with them on compassionate grounds but they wouldn't do it. I rang Qantas, the parent company of Jetstar but my pleas again fell on deaf ears. I didn't know it at the time but this is how businesses and organisations are these days. It's all about money and not about the people or customers at all. I was tired from the continuous fight I had endured in helping Leah and really couldn't be bothered fighting with a greedy company such as this. This sort of thing seemed so trivial at that moment. On that day I declared I would never fly Jetstar again, even though we had tens of thousands of frequent flier points. So I had to purchase two new tickets for the children to attend Leah's funeral. We headed to Melbourne for the service. Leah's parents had organised it all and allowed us to stay with them while we were down. I was so scatter brained that I forgot my suit pants and had to borrow a pair on the day. It was an extremely long morning as we readied ourselves for the funeral. Silence was still very prominent in Leah's parent's house as well. We went about our usual daily activities but with an empty feeling inside. But we had a funeral to attend. We went early to the chapel and the pure white casket was open for viewing. I had been strong throughout Leah's battle to give her and the children strength and confidence. But today was the day for the release of so much emotion, so many tears and so much grief. Leah looked peaceful. She had endured so much and now that was all behind her. She had peace. She was now free. The disgusting disease called cancer could do her no more harm. She could pass to the next place peacefully. She did look good. It was a blessing that she would be remembered looking so well and not like cancer had made her look at times. The service was amazing. The chapel had seating for about fifty guests. Fifty came and more followed. People kept arriving. The seats were taken. Standing room filled up. Guests spilled out into the street. It was huge. Hundreds turned up. I don't know how people heard of Leah's passing but friends I hadn't seen in many years were there. People I hadn't even met before, from Leah's childhood, turned up. She was such an adored person. We had been away for a few years but relationships had endured and now people wanted to come and say goodbye. I couldn't stop blubbering. I thought I would have to be strong for the children but this time I was not capable of doing this. I had lost the love of my life and it hurt so much. I hated this feeling. Would it ever go away? The children released a lot of grief as well. They had actually been so sure of the future that they hadn't really expressed much in the past. This day though was all about letting feelings show. The children stayed close by. They needed me that day more than ever. They would need me even more in the future. We, as a family, had a few years of frustration that came out that day. Terry, our neighbour from Hamilton Island, read out a children's book which Leah loved. This created more uncontrollable crying. The meaning and feeling of this book was multiplied many times over due to the event at which it was read. People couldn't contain the emotion. The grief in that little chapel was just too much. I had chosen the music for the service. Natalie Merchant featured. She is a great artist that I had loved for years and then Leah heard her songs and was hooked. Playing these beloved songs caused more grief. The music created such joyous memories. We had a slide show of photos from over the years. With all the traveling we had done we had collected so many photos and created so many memories. Small and insignificant moments now lost forever. These were milestones in our lives gone but not forgotten. Every direction I turned brought back amazing memories. Every person I looked at had been part of our history and each had a story or many stories. These stories flashed into my mind and created more agony. This was an exceptionally hard day. The minister asked if anyone wished to speak. I would have loved to but I was incapable. Others told me later that the same incapacitation had affected them. The service finished and we adjourned to the hotel for some reflection. The place was packed to the rafters with well wishers. Everyone had a story and such love and affection for Leah. That day was a fitting tribute to a woman who had been a part of so many lives and had left an indelible mark on so many people. People were in awe of Leah's bravery in the fight against cancer. Other qualities of Leah prior to cancer were also remembered. She was so bright and energetic. She had a real zest for life. I had never met a person with such vitality. I think that is why she was able to battle cancer so well. It was in her spirit. This was why so many wanted to be part of her life and wanted to be there to send her off so fittingly. The one consolation was, as everyone said, that Leah had lived an amazing life. Her forty years were filled with great memories. She had crammed so much into her life. Many would not have done half as much in their entire lives. This was a comforting thought at such a tragic time. She had two wonderful children, she had lived in paradise several times, she had travelled the world, had a Vegas wedding, met stars, had an amazing circle of friends, been on TV, radio and in the news, helped save lives, had a wonderful faith as a Christian and left a huge gap in so many lives due to her unique qualities that had inspired so many. It had been a special life that Leah had led. At her funeral that was celebrated well.

Our lives had changed forever. There were so many new things to work out. I had to establish our routines at home and I needed to find work. Ensuring that the children were fine was my first priority. Making sure I was alright as well. Who was I now? I became a widower. I became dad, a single dad. I was that guy who lost his wife. I think the day of Leah's death I lost my true identity. I felt like I didn't really belong. Ash had gone. I was now a gap filler. My role changed depending on the circumstance. I needed help. I would have liked a bit of time to ease into this new life. It wasn't the new life I had ever wanted or expected. Significant changes such as this take quite a lot of time to adapt and adjust to. But I didn't have that luxury. I was already getting reminders of our financial situation. This was to be the first situation I would need to attend to. The first solution was to be government assistance. I went to fill out all the forms to get the single parent pension. I had never been on benefits before and the process took ages. I rang to find out how to do it all. After what seemed an eternity on the telephone I was told I had to go to Lismore for interviews and to fill out the paperwork. I faced more traveling to Lismore? Great. I now hated the trip to Lismore. It contained so many bad memories. On some occasions I had to stop the car as something caused me to burst into tears. It may have been a song on the radio or a familiar landmark with wonderful memories. I felt alone at those moments. There were Centrelink, the government assistance organisation, offices closer but due to my circumstances I was required to attend the Lismore office. I needed the money so Lismore it was. The pension was a necessity until I could get back on my feet. I now had to pay for the debt left after trying to save my beloved. I had no job. My confidence was shot. Could I manage? Time would tell. The house was empty, the children were silent. We existed but after the children went to bed I had never felt so lonely. We had some counseling at the hospital. This had been priceless. I rang friends who gave me a shoulder to cry on. It took ages to get back to a state where I could even function. Don't get me wrong I could exist through habit. The kids got fed and managed to get to school and the day to day stuff just sort of happened but it was empty. I would hear something on the radio and laugh and couldn't wait to get home to tell Leah a funny story, but then reality would hit. The funny story suddenly became tragic, empty and worthless. A bit like how I felt. Leah had said, toward the end, how lucky she was knowing that the children had me if anything went wrong. Well things had gone terribly wrong, the children had me but that was of little comfort. What if something happened to me? That was another scenario I had to keep in the back of my mind. It was a frightening thought. I had to look after myself.

After some weeks survival became my instinct. It was hard. I had to start looking for work. I had mounting bills at high interest and they wouldn't just go away. I rang the bank and asked to see if they could refinance the medical debt onto my mortgage. They laughed. Our mortgage was about $1500 per month. It was cheaper than renting. But the money needed to service the other debt was over $2000 per month. This was impossible to pay in my situation. If I didn't pay, I got penalised. If I went over the limit I got another penalty. I tended to go over the limit quite often as I was right at the limit and couldn't reduce what I owed due to the expense. On a regular basis interest would be charged to my account and this would push me over the limit. I would therefore get another penalty charge. Even if it was just by 1 cent. I rang the banks and the accounts were cancelled. So it was just a matter of paying them back. But

I was still being charged an annual fee for having the accounts. The cheeky buggers.

I dealt with the financials during the day. After school the kids needed me. I had to be strong. They needed feeding. They needed clean clothes. Sometimes the food was two minute noodles. The clean clothes were occasionally what was worn that day, aired outside so at least they'd be fresh the next morning for school. The kids had trouble sleeping initially. Bim would ask to sleep in my bed. I missed someone in the bed so he was welcomed. Bec would often cry herself to sleep. Sometimes we would all fall asleep on the couch. We weren't physically tired but we were emotionally tired so often. This is how life went for quite some time.

So my main bank had laughed at me. I was tied to a number of banks so I would try the next one. Then the next one. Then the next. I was starting to worry. A few months had gone by since Leah's death and I was in a bit of a pickle. I did get some work but it was spasmodic. It wasn't substantial enough to help my refinance applications. None of it was full time. This was not the ideal position to be in when applying for finance. Being a single parent came with many predetermined stereotypical traits. It was hard to get things done or to avail services that I would have had ample opportunity to access over the past thirty years. This was a frustrating period in my life. Dealing with this and the rawness of the emotion after Leah's death was not a great experience. I tried logic. I sat down and wrote a letter to all the banks concerned. I set out to explain how I was in this situation. I explained Leah's journey. I mentioned the absence of help from Australia and the need to head overseas for treatment that worked amazingly. It was not like this was untested or an unrecognised treatment. It was available in hospitals all over the world. But not Australia. I used logic and reasoning in my communications with the banks. I used facts and figures. I pointed out the equity I had in the house. I questioned the ridiculous interest rates I was being charged. I pleaded that the rate of interest on my mortgage should be able to be applied to my entire debt. I explained the fact that by bundling all my debt together my monthly repayments would halve. I also used emotional reasoning. Our home was my wife's final resting place. The needs of the children were paramount and moving them would cause further devastation. I mentioned the availability of support from friends and neighbors' locally. I figured compassion might come into play. I then set about showing how if any of the banks took up this offer they would get more business, a happy customer and would enable me to halve my monthly expenses. I would take all my financial business to the bank that would respond to this offer. I sent this letter out and waited to see. While I was waiting for the banks to respond, life continued. The phone kept ringing. A lot of the calls were in relation to this treatment we had witnessed overseas. Of course I am not a doctor but people wanted information on how to access these treatments. They were desperate like we had been. For many it was a last option or a final chance. Shouldn't this type of thing be offered, if suitable, as one of the many options we were offered at the first diagnosis with any cancer? Shouldn't a doctor or oncologist be giving out information like this rather than the information coming from a single dad from country NSW? The other thing that intrigued me was that people thought this was new technology where as Cyberknife had been around for nearly a decade at the time and Gamma Knife nearly forty years but Australians had to find out by accident about it. I had so much going on at present but I remember our desperation during the search for help for Leah. I couldn't turn my back on these people asking for help. Many people were given a specific prognosis by their doctor. "You have six months to live." Or " There is nothing we can do." These words spoken by doctors brought back so many bad memories. Leah never wanted to know. It was irrelevant. Ian Gawler, who Leah had visited years before, was given six months to live. He is still alive and well over twenty years later. The prognosis given by doctors is given based on treatment options available in Australia. Many who have "inoperable" tumours could be treated by some of the overseas options. I felt it my duty to assist these people if I could. I was determined to change the lack of treatment options available for Australians and also to raise awareness of options available overseas, while we waited. I had been writing to Tony Abbott, who was our health minister at the time. I had been doing this since Leah's return from Oklahoma. He would respond on regular occasions and I was confident we were getting somewhere. Then Mr Abbott was coming to our region on a bike ride to raise awareness of prostate cancer. The local media decided to front Mr Abbott and ask how progress was going to get Cyberknife to Australia. He had no idea what they were talking about. This was frustrating. Obviously staff had vetted the correspondence I had been sending and it wasn't being passed on to the health minister. Then they were responding on his behalf. It was dishonest and a real slap in the face for people fighting cancer. I contacted the leader of the Democrats and she was excited by the prospect of Cyberknife. So she agreed to bring it up in Parliament as a question on notice to Mr Abbott. His response was both vague and non committal. I checked for other examples of this technology being discussed in Parliament. Surely the people with the power in this country were striving to ensure we were leaders in cancer care. There was not much but one great comment by a senator caught my eye.

He asked:

"I note that this cancer treatment is available in most countries overseas yet we don't have it in Australia. Can I ask? Are we the smartest country in the world and know something that all the other countries don't know and that is why we don't have these treatments and they do. Or are we the dumbest country in the world and the others the smartest as they are progressing and have these treatments?"

That's not word for word but pretty close and you get the sentiment, even if it was a bit sarcastic. This quote was also from notes made in 2004. The fact that 40,000 Australians die each year from cancer and they knew of this technology in 2004 but didn't do anything to get it was almost criminal. I mention this to people and they are disgusted. Armed with this type of information and attitude I knew this was going to be a tough but winnable battle. However, with the hurt and pain we had gone through, I was determined to try and prevent other families from going through the same. That was Leah's wish from a few years before. However I also felt that this was not the time to be devoting too much time to the cause of getting better cancer care to Australia. I had two kids who needed me. They both enjoyed the benefits of attending local schools. The teachers and fellow students helped so much. The routine involved in all aspects of school was vital in the children's wellbeing. After school we tried to do things as a family. It may have been as basic as just watching a movie together. I would be extra careful with Rebecca due to the house being dominated by boys. So we quite often watched a movie for her. Movies such as Sisterhood of the traveling pants and Elizabethtown come to mind. The first featured places like Santorini where Rebecca had been with Leah and I. The second, Elizabethtown, dealt with death and a quest to scatter the ashes of a loved one. You can well imagine that we would all end up sitting, watching and passing the tissues around. It was a bonding time. It was also a grieving time. We hadn't decided how we were going to approach dealing with scattering Leah's ashes and setting her free. It may have to wait till we got back on our feet financially. I wanted to take the kids to India and that would be an appropriate place as would Santorini. But these were thoughts for the future. We would keep Leah with us for the time being. We needed her close by. Leah's parents were devastated at this time as you can imagine, or perhaps not. We would try to support each other as best we could. The kids were a great help during this stage of all our lives. Leah's father and I had a love of plants and gardening. This interest helped as a diversion for the emptiness and hurt we were experiencing. They now had pretty empty lives. I really felt for them. No one should outlive their child. I endeavoured to maintain regular support with them and they reciprocated. It was imperative during our time of mourning. I would invite them up for Christmas and they would come. They'd stay a few days and enjoy festivities with the children and I. But there was always a tinge of sadness. Sometimes this was actually overwhelming sorrow. I hoped this was all part of the process of missing Leah. I was fortunate, in a sense, to be so busy with everything that these moments of utter grief were few. Late at night was the worst time. During the day I had distractions. This made it tolerable. Leah's parents had few distractions so the grief was quite debilitating. I tried to help from afar. Leah's mum decided on a holiday to San Diego to visit Jean, who Leah had met while having her Gamma Knife. This would be a great opportunity for both ladies to support each other and think of Leah. During this time Leah's dad came up and stayed with us for a few weeks. He didn't overly like the long flight so asked if we would put him up. Of course we said yes and this was a good break for both of them. I enjoyed the company of Leah's dad as he was a different person on his own and I felt like I had a new friend. I think the experience was good for him as well as it was a different scenario for him. They had never had separate holidays in all the time they'd been married.

But again, right through this time of mourning, I had been getting a number of enquiries about Cyberknife. I would relay our story and then tell them about a website which had videos, photo's, information, locations of Cyberknife around the world and contacts for patients. As I was still emotionally raw this was the easiest option for me and the most informative option for the person asking. The information could be gathered at the following website:

www.cyberknife.com

Some were asking as a last chance such as we had. Some were parents checking to see if their child was suitable, some were just refusing to go through the invasive options available in Australia and were willing to travel overseas and pay high costs to have a better chance and maintain quality of life. One lady rang to tell me about her story. She had just been diagnosed with cancer and the oncologist went to put her on chemotherapy the next week. She refused until she had researched it more. She found out about a test only available overseas which ascertains if chemotherapy would indeed be effective for her cancer, body type and the like. She had to travel to the USA for this test. It cost her about $6000 in airfares, accommodation and expenses but the result showed chemotherapy would not have worked for her. She would have been subjected to the side effects of this treatment with little result. So she declined chemotherapy and looked at other options.

While I was helping these people, amid our financial uncertainty, something amazing happened. A representative from the Australian government's department of Health and Ageing contacted me to pass on some information to a mother who had enquired about Cyberknife for her son. The Health department had heard of this and contacted me to pass on information about a funding program. MTOP is the Medical Treatment Overseas Program. It pays successful applicants, who are forced overseas if Australia doesn't have a suitable treatment here, their expenses. This includes two business class airfares for patient and carer, accommodation overseas, treatment and other expenses. This was amazing. No one had told us about this. I asked if we could apply retrospectively for this as the two treatments Leah had received had successfully treated her numerous tumours when no options were offered in Australia. The treatments had provided Leah a vast improvement in quality of life. They were successful and had cost us a fortune so I figured we were candidates for this funding. The only reason we had headed overseas was for the treatment of the brain which couldn't be done here. We hadn't needed to go overseas for any of the other cancer Leah had earlier as that was treatable here. But we had been forced to USA to obtain both Cyberknife and Gamma Knife due to the absence of any options in Australia for treating her brain tumours. In the end both treatments worked. It all sounded quite simple to me. We had other funding available in Australia for ailments that were self inflicted. Leah didn't ask for the brain tumours so I thought I would apply for MTOP funding. Was this the answer to our financial problems? I certainly hoped so. I filled out the application form. It didn't need much. Just notes from Leah's oncologist in Melbourne and the treating doctor in San Diego, as I was applying first for the Gamma Knife costs as they were more expensive than the Cyberknife and were first incurred. I had to provide a summary of why we went for Gamma Knife and any supporting evidence. That was it. I sent it off and waited. And waited. And waited. I would hate for this to be a matter of life and death. While all this was going on I figured I should create some sort of forum where all this information could be obtained easily. It would make it easier on me and provide more local information for the people asking for help. I set up the Facebook page called "Bring the Cyberknife cancer treatment to Australia". It got immediate responses. I had links to the company details of the people who make and supply the Cyberknife. I had links to the MTOP funding information and application. I added videos for people to view. I added politician details that people could use to contact them and ask for Cyberknife to be brought to Australia. I added patient stories. News articles, photo's, helpful information, a petition and all the hospital contact details where Cyberknife is available worldwide. Every day others added information or support as well. We quickly got thousands of signatures on the petition. People were frustrated with the lack of options in Australia. People wanted to forgo the invasive and debilitating treatment options currently available in Australia for something gentler and a lot quicker. Many, as Leah had mentioned in her final months, would quite happily have used a less invasive treatment and avoid the associated side effects of what was currently available in Australia. They would have used something like Cyberknife, even if the end result was still to be the same. Quality of life was so important to many during treatment and after. Leah had felt that if the end result for her was still death then she would have preferred less treatment, more quality of life in those years, more time with her family and more time away from hospitals and doctors. Cyberknife and Gamma Knife could have allowed that if it were available anywhere in Australia. The other thing I did at this time was to set up a Facebook page for Rebecca. She was spending a lot of time discovering interests away from us as a family. I took this to heart but was assured by friends that this was what teenagers did. She preferred to get her support from her friends, most being female. I knew she missed the female influence around home. My teenage years were too far away in my memory to compare. But Rebecca's seclusion was a positive time for her. She delved into reading huge novels and also painting which Leah loved and was so good at. The Facebook site I developed was a gallery of some of Rebecca and Leah's artwork. It allowed people from all over the world to reflect on some of Leah's past art and also to watch Rebecca develop in this area. I was very proud of both of them. If you go to Facebook and search for Rebecca and Leah's art gallery you can see some of this wonderful work.

Another thing I noted, which really upset me during these times, was that everyone else was able to resume life as normal. The grief was still there but the day to day events went back to normal. They were able to mourn the loss of Leah from their lives in a comfortable environment and at their own pace. We weren't able to do that. We cried, we mourned and we ached but had to do it under duress. I don't feel this did justice to Leah. It certainly made it difficult and frustrating for us. The banks didn't ease up. It wasn't fair for me or the children to not have a proper transitional period after Leah's death. We were all still so sad. However we were forced to make concessions in the manner and time we put in to our mourning. That is something we will never get back.

# Chapter 20

# Channel seven and Leahbelles via Byron Bay

Life was very difficult for all of us during this time. Our wonderful life had come crashing down around us. The one saving grace was the ability to help others. We were beginning to get a great deal of exposure with the local news, letters to the editor in the paper and on radio. We then got an unexpected ally in the fight to get Cyberknife to Australia. I got a phone call from a man at Channel seven television here in Australia. They wanted to do a story on Cyberknife to increase the chances of getting it to Australia. This man's younger brother had a brain tumour and was offered no choices in Australia. His family was forced to look to The Netherlands in an attempt to help this young 17 year old boy beat cancer. So the man from Channel seven was very keen to do a story and raise awareness of the state of the art treatment that Australians were being denied access to unless they were able to travel overseas to get it. I was the one who had already had significant publicity so he asked if he could set up an interview. I agreed but was just at the beginning of starting a new business to help with the financial strain we were experiencing. They were very flexible and agreed to fit it in around my schedule. I was more than happy to oblige.

I had been a TAFE teacher in Melbourne and also during my time on Hamilton Island. So I approached the closest college to our home to enquire about work. I had left my resume and waited. I had picked up little bits of work here and there but many wanted me to work nights. The children were too young and had just lost their mum so I didn't want to work nights and leave them vulnerable. They needed a parent around. I needed to be there for them. But I also needed something concrete in the way of regular income. I was starting to worry. I was looking for meaningful work but wasn't getting anything secure or steady. I needed security at present as I could feel everything slipping away. I was looking as far as Robina on the Gold Coast which was over one hour away. I even applied for some work in Brisbane which would have been about three hours away in peak hour. These were full time jobs which would have helped my applications with the banks to allow me to consolidate my high interest debt into my low interest mortgage. Many of these potential employers declined my application due to the distance and the fact I was a single parent.

I needed to catch a break. But I didn't think I could rely on others. I had to make things happen for myself. So I decided to open up part of the house as a bed and breakfast. People loved when we entertained so why not use this strength and get the work to come to us rather than me chasing it. I set it all up. I decided that I would take just one couple at a time. I would cater to their every whim. I decided to personalise each guests stay. I would cook their meals. I wanted to make them feel welcome and not want to leave. Taking just one couple at a time would also make it a manageable venture. The room we set up had glass on two walls. This overlooked the rainforest over to the coast. It was magical. The same two sides had a wonderful verandah that people could laze about on to help relax and they could even have meals out there. I put in a huge glass door in the bathroom and this looked out over the rainforest as well. As we had no neighbours on that side, or very close at all actually, guests would be able to sit in the bath, have some champagne and relax while looking out over the rainforest. It became a wonderful little spot for people to visit. I had set it up ready to go but couldn't decide on a name. We were near Byron Bay and I wanted to use Byron Bay in the name so when people did a search we would show up in the Byron Bay enquiries. Byron B and B, Byron Hinterland, Byron Tree tops and Byron Rainforest Retreat. I couldn't decide on one and they all seemed quite impersonal. Then an amazing thing happened. Lots of coincidences had happened in my life. Another one happened at this time. A friend rang one night to check up on us. Whenever Caz used to ring for Leah she would ask for Leahbelle. She was the only one who referred to Leah by this name. As we reminisced she referred to Leah as Leahbelle quite a few times and I liked the name. It sounded appropriate, so the bed and breakfast became known as Leahbelles. I called it Leahbelles via Byron Bay on websites and cards. All the requirements of a name were met. It was a lovely touch to mark Leah's final home and for her to be part of the solution I needed to get back on my feet. I had a website set up, got some cards printed and we opened for our first booking on Valentine's day (ironic in a way as Leah had been initially diagnosed with breast cancer on a Valentine's day many years previously). I feel Leah may have been looking down with approval on us and that's why this date was to see our first booking. This business would enable me to still pick up little odd jobs, be there for the children and if I had to work nights it would be from home. Leah and I had joked about not setting up a hospitality business as it would mean working seven days a week and all the responsibility and paperwork but it was now necessary to do this to avoid losing the lot. This was another twist in the new direction our lives were taking.

Bookings flowed and it was a pleasurable way to make a living. I couldn't save any money as it all went on the mortgage and the huge medical debt still owed but at least I was keeping my head above water. The children could remain in school locally and I was able to get some scraps of work on top of the bed and breakfast income. I loved that people arrived as guests and left as friends. I had one couple from Brisbane who stayed on five different occasions and loved our proximity to them and the pampering they got from us. Even the kids got involved. Bim received a $10 tip from this customer for bringing a bowl of ice for their drinks. Bloody expensive ice I joked. This experience was also great for our healing. Having mum involved in the future in the form of a bed and breakfast was fitting. We wanted to remember Leah and have her in our lives even though she was gone from us. Our guests enjoyed this aspect of the business as well.


We were on 10 acres. It was surrounded by rainforest and a small stream. We had 3 alpacas which were used to keep the grass down. I loved gardening so I planted a vast array of fruit, vegetables and flowers to help make the bed and breakfast experience unique. I would put beautiful dragon fruit on the breakfast platter. Not many had experienced this so it was a great way to surprise guests. I added our lemon myrtle and local honey to yoghurt so guests could spoon this on muesli with home grown goji berries. We had mangoes and passionfruit. I was growing pomegranates and sopote. I even planted an apple tree. People said I was mad and that it was too hot and humid to grow. But I had a shady side of a hill that suited the apple tree perfectly. I grew blue berries and strawberries. We even had some banana trees. I was able to grow kipfler potatoes, snow peas, carrots and pumpkins just sprung up everywhere. In the summer it was tomatoes and I grew corn and a vast array of unusual herbs. I had a kaffir lime tree, lemongrass and coriander. It was truly breathtaking to be able to wander around the property and pick produce we had grown. If I ran short then the produce in town was grown by people we knew anyway. My customers loved seeing their food grow before their eyes. So it hadn't taken much to be ready for business and now the television crew was coming to do an interview.

So now the people Channel seven were coming to visit our wonderful home. They confirmed the date of when they would come and do an interview. The lovely reporter, Marguerite McKinnon, and her camera and sound guys came up from Sydney. They did a bit of background questioning and the interview went ahead. No one involved in the filming had ever heard of Cyberknife. This was not unusual in Australia. I showed scans that the doctors had done of Leah's brain to ensure the Cyberknife was accurate. I had a vast file of information including brochures, video of Leah getting the treatment and patient information sheets. They asked about the children. They asked how they were coping with the loss of their mum and they made enquiries as to how I was paying for the expense of all the cancer care. That last one was hard to answer as it seemed like I was taking one step forward and then two steps back. They were very compassionate throughout the entire process and I actually enjoyed the experience. The children had a few shots taken of them around the house and Marguerite took the videos of Leah to edit it all into a story they hoped would make a difference. When I told them about the bed and breakfast they wanted to have a look. Then they decided on taking some footage for the story so I could get some publicity and assist with getting extra business. They really were wonderful people. They had spent most of the day with us. The actual story was only going to be about 10 minutes long. They took a wealth of information with them when they went. We couldn't wait to see the finished story on the actual show on television when it was to be shown. We only had to wait a few days for it to air. The television show was Today Tonight. We watched it on the night we were featured. Today Tonight had incorporated Patrick Swayze into the piece as he was undergoing Cyberknife in USA at the same time our story was done. This was another bizarre twist in this tale. Patrick had pancreatic cancer which is a real nasty one. They only expected him to last a month or so. He was having Cyberknife along with chemotherapy. He was filming a movie at the time and he lasted months more than expected. This allowed Patrick to finish his filming. So Channel seven opened the Today Tonight show with images of Patrick Swayze and dirty dancing. This brought back many memories of the time he had danced passed us in Los Angeles. Then they interviewed some patients from the USA and then on to us. They had edited images and footage of Leah into the segment and it was like she was still here. It was uncanny but fitting that Leah could still be involved in helping others by raising awareness of the life saving treatment called Cyberknife. The segment was also put onto the Today Tonight website to allow people to access it further at a later stage if they missed it or to get any contact details. They had interviewed a doctor from a Sydney hospital for his opinion and he was obviously suitably impressed. His contact details were also available on the website. They had done a nice segment on Leahbelles and then included our contact details on the Channel seven website as well. It was a very successful show and the response was amazing. The Channel seven switchboard went into meltdown and so did my phone. After that show I got about a hundred calls or emails a day. Some people rang to offer us condolences. Others were angry at the people who can make a difference in Australia but actually weren't. Others wanted to book the bed and breakfast. Others contacted me with offers to help gain exposure for Cyberknife. Many rang for help with getting the treatment and were amazed at how many hospitals had it worldwide. Some went ahead with obtaining the Cyberknife in USA or Malaysia or Turkey. It got a bit tiresome going over the details of Leah's illness and associated adventures but I never shirked what I thought was my responsibility. This was a way of assisting others to at least have Cyberknife as an option in their battle against cancer. The interest and enquiries slowed as time passed but I still got several contacts a day and still do to this day. It showed people have a huge interest in anything different to what was being dished up as the only options in cancer treatment at the time.

The process of helping others was quite therapeutic for me as well. Rather than holding everything in I was able to talk about our loss and this helped me cope with Leah's death. The compassion shown by others was also very comforting for the children.

I was running my bed and breakfast, looking after the children, doing odd bits and pieces of casual work and now dealing with an influx of requests for help with people's cancer choices. While all this was going on I figured I should update my forum where all this information could be obtained easily. I amended my Facebook page called "Bring the Cyberknife cancer treatment to Australia". It was getting a huge response again due to the television exposure. We soon had 5000 supporters. People found out via this site about MTOP funding which made the choice a lot easier to make. Some would ring and thank me when they were accepted for this funding. I was still, however, waiting for my approval for Leah's trips. Just about every day others added information to this support site as well. I had a number of doctors join up to assist and also patients from overseas and Australia who had undergone the Cyberknife treatment. As Cyberknife was available worldwide in about 200 hospitals my page was well received and supported and before long we had thousands of people joining the fight. Letters were sent to the health minister, at the time Tony Abbott and then after a federal election, to Nicola Roxon who took over the portfolio of health. The word was getting around about this treatment and people contacted me who had gone overseas to get the Cyberknife for themselves. This enabled me to gather a serious amount of information to assist people enquiring. It also enabled people to support us by contacting the appropriate people in government, health and media to try and get Cyberknife to Australia. The support by the media, in many forms, also grew as a result of the story done by Channel seven. I had opened myself up to public scrutiny but if this helped fulfill Leah's wish to help others then it was well worth it. She had said that if all this saved just one life, stopped one family going through what we were forced to endure then this would all be worth it. When I got the first visit from someone who had been saved by Cyberknife, after all options had been exhausted in Australia, I was overcome with emotion. We all broke down into tears of relief, joy and a tinge of sadness. Relief that we were seeing results in Australia of Cyberknife. Joy, as at least one life had been saved. Leah was gone but my effort in her memory enabled others to live. We also felt sadness in the fact that we found out about Cyberknife too late for Leah. Her body had been through too much to endure and, in the end, it gave up after an amazing fight. Sadness too for many people who would die not knowing what was available out there. Some of these people may have benefitted from Cyberknife. We also felt sadness for families that, even if they did know of Cyberknife, may not have been able to travel to access it. Cancer is a disease that creates this sort of conflict of emotions. Our first day, that Valentine's day so many years ago was filled with some of the greatest highs and the most devastating low as well. These emotions still had a huge impact on our lives today.

# Chapter 21

# Ebay, Kyle and Jackie O

My biggest issue at this stage was that I still hadn't been able to obtain a refinance from any bank to consolidate this high interest medical debt. Interest was up to 25%. I was only paying interest and no principal as that was all I could afford. Any fees or charges, and there were plenty, took the principal higher and I ended up going backwards. I hated the absolute waste of money. Money I could have used for my kids. I hadn't been too concerned up to this point as I was able to juggle the money around to get by up to now. But soon I was running low on the available funds that had helped me balance this financial juggling act. The funds I was using to juggle with were in the form of a small window of credit within each debt. I could use this credit in the short term to pay other banks. This created a window with that bank which made it possible to use that small amount of equity to pay yet another bank and so on. Not an ideal way to exist, and that's just what it was, existing. But until a refinance or the MTOP funding came my way it would have to do. I had been with ANZ for over twenty years and had some of this debt with them so I applied with them at one stage. This provided the first breakthrough with this entire mess. The loan was approved but with certain criteria. The main requirement was that all the high interest debt would be eradicated and then I would have only the one mortgage which would be easily managed. My problem appeared solved. Everyone would be happy. ANZ got a happy client and some extra business. The other banks were to get their money repaid and I could begin to start a new life unencumbered by this ridiculous debt hanging over my head. The representative of the ANZ walked me through each stage and was able to approve the amount I needed based on my income which was starting to become more regular. It was tight. The loan approval was just on the limit. But that's all I needed. The loan was approved and just had to settle and I could start budgeting like a normal family again. Well that's what I thought was going to happen. The process of getting this loan took five months. I was studying at college to update my teaching qualifications at the time. I was on a lunch break at college when my current mortgage provider rang me to tell me I had missed a payment on my mortgage. I explained that I no longer had a mortgage with them due to the ANZ loan settling that day. I was then informed that the settlement never went ahead. That was it. No explanation, no compassion, just another fee charged to me for late payment. My heart sank, not for the first time. I was in class so would have to wait until later to respond to all concerned. It is lucky that I am a patient man. But my patience was wearing a bit thin by now. When I got home I rang ANZ to find out what the hell had gone wrong after five months of absolute compliance on my behalf. I was told that due to the addition of interest and penalties and charges over the five month period that the amount I had been approved to borrow was insufficient to clear the total debt by a few thousand dollars. As mentioned earlier, the requirement for the loan approval was that all my unsecured debt was paid out by the ANZ loan. However due to these charges the amount I would need to clear my debt was now slightly higher. The amount that I'd applied for and was approved for was now insufficient to meet the terms of the new loan. My new life changing mortgage would not proceed. Instead of going ahead with the loan based on the figures from five months ago and leaving me a small amount of higher interest debt , ANZ had pulled out of the entire deal. The settlement of the new loan would not proceed. I was back at square one. But I was actually now worse off. I pleaded with them to make the loan go ahead and leave me with the small amount of higher interest debt as I would be able to cope with that small amount quite easily. They declined. So after many months of battling to get my finances consolidated to make it manageable I was worse off now than ever. Of course the costs involved in getting the loan would still need to be paid. Each time I went for a loan I had to get a new valuation on the house. These cost about $600 each. The costs were mounting. Still, I figured I had gotten close with the ANZ and I was sure to get the MTOP funding so that would reduce the amount I needed to refinance. Things would shortly turn the corner. But in the meantime I still had to deal with the ANZ phone calls demanding payment on time and threatening me if I was late or over the limit. I was amazed at the lack of communication and also the lack of understanding and flexibility by them.

However just as I thought things wouldn't or couldn't get any worse I got notification from the Health department that my application for MTOP funding had been declined. Now things were starting to get a bit more serious. How was I going to manage all of this? I had developed a great little business in Leahbelles. The children were firmly entrenched in their wonderful little lives. But how could I pay for all of this in any logical manner. Every mainstream avenue I turned to was letting me down. The banks had refused to assist me and the government had turned its back on us as well. It felt like it was the kids and I against the world. I tried to shelter the children, as much as I could, against the severity of our financial situation. It was very much one day at a time. We couldn't plan, we couldn't organise anything more than a few days away. We were lucky to live where we did as there was so much natural beauty around for the children to enjoy. The many families that lived nearby were very helpful as well. We didn't need much money really to survive. This was just as well. I was able to grow a lot of our own food. Fruit and vegetables in the garden grew well. Our water was free as we had rain water tanks and a spring fed dam. We needed small wardrobes of clothes as we had few formal occasions to dress up for. We spent time together and enjoyed movies at home, our favourite television shows and games around the property. Our life could have been idyllic except for this rotten debt. The fight was going to be tough. How to win it when the well was almost empty was the big question. My confidence was at an all time low. I had been so strong when helping Leah as we would see results and have huge breakthroughs and wins. This wasn't happening any more. The process of applying for loans and funding was exhausting as well. The phone calls were tiresome and demanding. I felt worthless, had no money and was really struggling emotionally. What was left that I could do?

Ebay became the answer. I went through the house and found old kids toys, plants out of the garden and I even put gift vouchers for Leahbelles up for sale. I would dig beautiful Heliconias out of our garden, divide them and list them on Ebay. I sold the children's collection of Beanie Kids. They had over 350. They wanted me to have them and sell them. This was heart breaking. As I was going through things in the house to sell I came upon Leah's cancer stuff. Her Cyberknife scans were in the file. They had cost us about $1000 each at the time and there were about a dozen of them so I thought I would auction them. It would raise awareness of our plight while also getting information out there about Cyberknife. I scanned a photograph of the Cyberknife scan, wrote a little story about why they were for sale and I listed them. I had a few nibbles, the scans got featured in local media but it was slow going. Then a major newspaper writer approached me. She wrote a story on my situation which generated about 100 replies. Some people wrote showing support for us and many were shocked by the lack of help for us. But others put me in touch with legal services, financial advisers and the like. The response and concern was quite overwhelming. Some of these people suggested bankruptcy. It would leave us homeless but eradicate the debt. Could a bankrupt single dad of two even get a rental property if I was to do that? I doubt it. I didn't like that idea anyway. I had always paid my way. A couple of other financial advisers suggested against declaring bankrupt. I would prefer not to. I had worked all my life and never shirked a debt and didn't feel like doing so now either. The journalist also suggested rather than selling the actual scans that I could sell a copy of the scan for just a few dollars and then email the copy to the buyer. This was a great idea and I implemented it straight away. Again it created numerous sales and a lot of interest in the Cyberknife. A lady from the Macquarie University in Sydney even contacted me to ask if I'd consider putting the Cyberknife scans in an exhibition being put together by the great auction house, Sotheby's. I was very excited by this offer and accepted. The exhibition was of a range of modern day diverse objects of interest. This exhibition had around sixty items ranging from jewellery, vases, toys and statues. This was a quirky little twist in our ever changing story. However even with these additional sources of income it soon became apparent that a few hundred dollars here or there actually didn't help. The debt itself could be quite manageable but how it was structured meant that I needed to pay huge chunks off it at a time to make any inroads. This was rarely possible so it hardly ever changed for the positive and quite often I went backwards. The other thing the journalist suggested, after asking what else I had available to sell, was quite shocking. I told her that just about everything we had that we didn't need or use was already up for sale. I had sold half of the garden, kids toys and clothes, my shirts and shoes. Sarcastically, I said just about the only thing left was Leah's ashes. She fell silent and told me she'd ring me back. She actually did some investigating and got back to me with the suggestion of listing Leah's ashes for sale on Ebay. I was shocked. I felt sick to the stomach that someone would even suggest this. I was utterly devastated to even be having the conversation. Was I really in that much of a pickle? She persisted, gently. She explained to me that she had researched this the day before. She told me that it was actually not possible to sell the ashes but that I could list them, create awareness of the ridiculous situation we were in and that before they could sell, Ebay would remove the ashes from the site due to a contravention of their rules. Publicity would be generated and there would be no risk of actually losing Leah's ashes. She even remarked that, in a funny way, Leah would be contributing to the solution. She felt that this may create a situation where someone may even offer to help us out. Maybe a private investor would refinance our property at a logical interest rate. She thought that maybe we may get some donations from generous people. Maybe we could sell our story. Who knows? Obviously I baulked at the idea. I cried. I was scared. This realisation, of the state I was actually in, had really shocked me more than at any stage before. I felt extremely alone again. What had my life come to? How could such an amazing life suddenly free fall out of control so quickly? Surely there must be a fair solution rather than this route? However the banks kept ringing. They were relentless. Sometimes Bim would answer the phone, pass it to me horrified and I would have to deal with a late payment, over limit or whatever else they were harassing me for. I would quite often end up in tears of frustration. They were tears of sadness and frustration. Bim was not exactly sure what was going on but he didn't like the effect it would have on me. I would tell the banks that I'd written to them with a solution. The representatives I would speak to were quite often sympathetic. Some even shared my tears. But in the end they would tell me it was their job to ring and that I needed to make a payment or risk defaulting. I would end the phone calls very frustrated and quite upset. Bim was great and would curl up on the couch with me for a hug. He was only six years old when this all started so he didn't really understand what it was all about. But you don't need a reason for a hug. The banks couldn't take that away from us. But I also knew I needed to do something very quickly. I was working two or three jobs and getting nowhere fast. I actually then contemplated listing Leah's ashes for sale. I hesitated and dwelled on this for some time but then decided I had no alternative. So I did it. I listed the ashes on Ebay.

The journalist who suggested I list Leah's ashes was right. I got a huge response. I was featured on numerous radio programs. I had a couple of TV networks interested and the printed media as well. I was still at college studying at the time. My phone went off the hook during classes. People wanted to interview me. This was a chance to get my message of injustice out there. I made a few appointments for interviews. ABC radio wanted to know why I would do such a thing as list my late wife's ashes. I explained and they wanted answers from the banks and the government as well. People would ring in and offer consolation which was comforting. It was the beginning of a range of different topics which were taken up by some of these media outlets. I continued to get great support from the ABC. They had been very supportive of the quest to get Cyberknife to Australia. They were interested in my story as well. I built some great relationships with the staff at ABC. Kyle and Jackie O from 2Day FM in Sydney were in London and they had heard of our story. They wanted to interview me from the UK. They had a huge following as they were one of the top rating radio shows in Sydney at the time. The producer assured me that it would be a sympathetic interview. I agreed to do it and began to plan the range of topics to discuss. I wanted to talk about the cancer treatments not available to Australians and the cost of heading overseas for the treatments. I also wanted to touch on the discrimination against patients unable to travel or who couldn't afford to. I wrote a list of topics I wanted to discuss with them on the radio. This was my big chance to change everything. However the segment on the Kyle and Jackie O show was more of a set up. They introduced me but didn't let me get much of a defense or explanation across about our situation. They just launched into the story of a man selling his wife's ashes. Then they transferred me to a group of handpicked angry callers who were upset with me listing Leah's ashes. I was then expected to defend myself which would apparently make for entertaining radio. Jackie was actually quite sympathetic and compassionate which was touching. However after the segment aired the producers would not respond to me ever again. I had been dumped. I had served my purpose. They had a link on the 2Day FM website about my guest spot which people actually responded to. I wrote on here to give my side of the story. Many of the responses on this site were supportive and understanding. This posts on the website were different responses to those of the listeners who were selected for the on air interview earlier. After just a few hours this link was deleted by the radio station. I was again left on my own. This was a sensation I was feeling a lot of lately. The banks had a knack of making me feel the same way. Now a radio station had done it also but in the most public of forums. I felt humiliated and double crossed. I was at my lowest ever. I don't listen to 2Day FM anymore even though they have some of my favourite announcers such as Hamish and Andy.

A number of newspapers wanted a story and two television stations came out to cover the story as well. By the time all this happened, just over two days, the ashes had been pulled off the site by Ebay. The original journalist was right about the fact that the ashes would never get the chance to sell. This was the one consolation at this time. They had only been on the site for such a short time. This had been a huge relief and the stress I felt for that short time abated somewhat. I hadn't been able to eat or sleep. I was a wreck. Now after the radio debacle my nerves were shot. I was at my lowest. Bad thoughts entered my mind. I was beginning to think there was not any light at the end of the tunnel. These thoughts subsided when I saw my kids. They were keeping me alive. I had never any intention of selling the ashes but it was a desperate measure I needed to take to try and get some action on a number of issues which were just being swept under the carpet by those involved. I may have had no intention of selling the ashes but people who heard the story didn't know that. That is part of the reason I wrote this story. To fill in the gaps. I could see how demoralising the media could be. They can use people as pawns in the quest to boost ratings. I just wished they were skillful enough to entertain rather than taking the lazy option which is what they did with me. I have seen so many examples of this style of presenting on radio and feel it is very irresponsible. However the majority of the journalists I had dealt with were professional and skilled so I shouldn't tar them all with the one brush. It is a small minority who lack the ability to be successful on their own merits. It's funny that they all tend to be on the one radio network.

A few days after listing Leah's ashes on Ebay they were back in our arms. After this episode some of the media assisted me in getting my side of the story across but not everyone heard it. So some people continued with their misconception of the entire episode. Some of these people were family. Many phone calls were made to clarify the situation. Many of these people were in our local community. The story actually reached as far away as Europe so it is little wonder that it had created quite a stir. It even made it quite high within our government. Some of the journalists who covered the story wanted to talk with Nicola Roxon. She was the federal health minister at the time. Her department administered the MTOP funding scheme I had applied for to cover the costs of Leah's treatment in USA. She declined to speak to the media. I was not surprised there. But her silence created a bit more Interest by the media. Other journalists took an interest in the cancer treatment and wondered why we didn't have it in

Australia. They made some enquiries and then did further stories on it. Some even spoke with cancer experts overseas to get a further understanding of all the considerations needed to be taken into account about Cyberknife. The ABC followed up with further story into Cyberknife and used it in a positive manner to help with the effort of getting the treatment to Australia. They interviewed experts in the USA to obtain doctors opinions of the effectiveness of Cyberknife. This was really well researched and produced. I was glad to see some positive outcome from this horrendous situation. Then they did quite a comprehensive segment on Cyberknife and interviewed me as well as the practitioners overseas using Cyberknife. My faith in the media had been restored. The journalists at the ABC were professional, compassionate and genuinely wanted to help. They were journalists not shock jocks. The story was also put onto the ABC website and is still available today. Many people gathered new information from that segment to assist in their research into cancer care options. That's what we had wanted. That's what Leah had wanted.

Leah's ashes had 150 enquiries prior to being removed due to contravention of Ebay listing rules. Leah would have laughed. She had a great sense of humour. I also had a good sense of humour but just felt like crying. This wasn't funny for me. I had the debt. No denying that. However the debt was only created due to the fact that I loved Leah so much. So much, that I was forced to send her to the other side of the world for a treatment that may have saved her life. But that was a cost I was only too willing to take on. Leah had felt a little guilty of the cost but I assured her not to worry. After all it worked. She only ever mentioned her concern of the cost once. I think she could see my genuine desire to get her well. Life was the only factor to consider. Money comes and goes but we only get one chance of life. She was satisfied with my explanations and her silly concerns about the money dissipated. Yet now I had been made to feel second rate, worthless and almost like a criminal due to seeking this world class care for a loved one. I was now virtually prostituting myself to the media in order to survive. I felt worthless, dirty and a shadow of my former self. I had no confidence any more. Yet the manner in which I sought help for Leah was done out of love, generosity and a desire to help. That desire to help still existed. My children needed and deserved a normal childhood. This I tried to provide. But during this phase of our lives I was also encountering numerous new emotions and sensations that I was not happy feeling. I must say that cost had never been an issue with any of the decisions we made in the pursuit of Leah's health. We had previously received assistance from friends or family. The cost of this treatment had nothing to do with Leah. It was an action we had to take. It was the only option. Why should she feel guilty? If these treatments had been available in Australia we would have had immediate access to them and the result may have been different. We are the ones who should feel guilty for denying sick people in Australia these recognised treatment options. When any negative thoughts entered my mind I was able to reflect on the wonderful and generous people we had encountered during this cancer journey. This helped me face the continuous stream of demands made by the banks during this time. It didn't make it go away but it ensured I was able to step back and see it for what it really was.

We got a lot of exposure by doing something that still weighs heavily on my mind and in my heart. I was beginning to question the saying that Australia is the lucky country. We are so far behind with cancer care options. We are ignored when our social status changes. We are denied funding for something that does exactly what the funding asks the treatment to do. People are forced into ridiculous situations just to provide for their family. I knew I was not alone. People throughout the world struggled with injustices every day. Many were in more dire situations than mine. But my late mother had instilled in me the trait of persistence. I was definitely not giving up, even though I came very close a couple of times. Luckily the ashes didn't sell. It had been such a difficult situation to go through. I had done everything within my power to raise some awareness of our situation without risking such a prized possession of my family's. Even the photo I used on the Ebay listing was of a "memory bottle". Our friend Terry had given this bottle to us, upon Leah's death, so we could always have lovely memories of Leah. I had used this in the Ebay photo rather than the actual urn holding Leah's ashes. I had to draw the line somewhere. As well as Europe, the story ended up being featured in many places around the world. USA, UK and others. We had been in the news for such a bizarre reason. What had started out as a quest to save a beautiful woman by going overseas, to the USA, for a treatment not available to Australians, had now created news, around the world, of us back in Australia trying to battle bureaucracy as a result of the costs involved. We were not provided with any options at the time. We were still being denied options. I was really starting to feel like I was sinking fast. How long could this go on? I got a great deal of exposure from this episode in my life. Some was supportive. Others, including family and friends, were quite disgusted in my actions. I don't blame them. But they didn't know the full story. But we also didn't receive any suggestions of a solution. Someone suggested I get another job. But I had three going as it was. Some suggested financial planning or an adviser but I had already done that and the result kept coming up the same. I got abused. I got offers of assistance in kind. Even though the episode generated quite a lot of exposure to our plight, a solution still didn't come from it. We were still treading water. At least my list of media contacts had grown. That was about the only consolation out of the whole forgettable experience.

One really upsetting situation came up during this time. After our trip to India we had sponsored three children from overseas. It was lovely getting updates on their progress from time to time. I felt it to be a rewarding experience for the children. However now times were tough. I couldn't afford this "luxury" any more. So I rang up to cancel. But it's not that simple. I was given a period of time to see if my circumstances would improve and then I could continue on. I had to agree to this because if I said my circumstances wouldn't improve, I would be admitting defeat. So in a few months I would get a call and go through the process again. I have still not been able to continue on with this sponsorship even after several years but I hope to one day.

# Chapter 22

# An appealing situation

I was amazed at how well the children had adjusted to our new life that we had been thrust into upon Leah's death. It had taken a while but as a family we dealt with the grief as best we could and now we were learning to live our new lives. A lot of the time it wasn't pleasant but it was a necessity of life. The kids used to go to bed crying in the early days. It took ages for this to subside. I would often cry myself to sleep as well. Some nights I wasn't sure of the reason I was crying. I was very confused in those early days. Rebecca had pleaded with me at the time not to uproot the family and move. We hadn't and to see them heal in this beautiful environment in which we lived was reward enough for my promise to Rebecca. I had done everything I could to keep the family together in our family home. We were surrounded by memories of Leah. Her black and white cows adorned a whole wall. Her other mosaics were scattered around the property. A wonderful magnolia planted as a memorial grew next to a pond I built from rocks dug out of the ground. In this environment the children were allowed to develop. We had wonderful neighbours and dear friends who assisted us every day and also helped with the healing. We all remembered Leah fondly on many regular occasions. Anniversaries were the worst but we tried to celebrate rather than commiserate. Most of the time our financial problems were in the background rather than the focus of our lives but at times it was difficult.

I had been denied funding through the medical treatment overseas program (MTOP) and a solicitor had been made aware of our situation through the news stories about our ashes sale. The solicitor rang me and offered to assist in submitting an appeal against the health department's decision to deny the funding. I was feeling quite tired and quite helpless at the moment so a ray of light, such as this, was extremely welcome. I took all the information I had to the solicitor and he was amazed. From the first instance he looked at Leah's medical records, scans and x rays, history and treatments he was convinced that the government was wrong. He hung on to the file I had brought him and made some enquiries himself. He was quite thorough and gave more substance to what I had been saying all along. He got expert testimony from USA and Europe. He thought this important as they were countries using the technology. Australia did not have it yet it was Australians making the decision. As the MTOP decision was made by Australian and New Zealand "experts" that didn't have or use the technology that Leah sought, the solicitor felt that this was vital in the case. He wondered how they could make a decision when we don't even have these treatments in this country. Hospitals using these technologies overseas obviously have records of the treatments and statistics on the outcomes. The Australian experts deciding our fate based the outcome on reports dating back over four years at the time. The statistics used in this country are quite dated and this technology advances so rapidly that unless we were actually using the treatments here a valid conclusion could not be made. Well this is what the solicitor told me. He was the expert in his field. He was amazed at the wealth of knowledge that was available but had not been used in determining my outcome. The treatment, Gamma Knife had been around since 1968. It had treated millions of patients. Gamma Knife was available worldwide. It was actually the treatment of choice for the exact cancer Leah had. The other aspect that irritated my solicitor was the fact that the decision was made after Leah had passed away. The criteria for deciding on the appropriateness of the funding should be made before the treatment was sought. We didn't know of the funding prior to Leah's trip so this was now impossible. The solicitor stated, in part of his appeal, that they must make the decision based on a retrospective application and not use information associated with Leah's death. Based on other cases we knew of, Leah's case being looked at retrospectively should have been successful. We knew of people who had gone overseas for treatments with other ailments as well as the cancer and been successful in obtaining the funding. Based on this, Leah's was straight forward, apparently. The other thing the solicitor mentioned was that the criteria used for assessing eligibility was extremely broad. This had to be positive for our case as it allowed for a fair amount of interpretation. Here is a list of the four criteria we had to meet:

1. The treatment or similar must not be available in Australia.

We had enquired and been given no treatments in Australia as options. We have stereotactic radio surgery devices but not as advanced as what is on offer overseas. If we did, don't you think we would have avoided the stress of travel, overseas support and other inconveniences of seeking treatment elsewhere? They said we had similar treatments here and so denied us this eligibility criterion. It is ironic though. As I write this a Sydney hospital have just started using its first Gamma Knife machine. Why would we need it here if the government feels we already have suitable treatments? I think they had contradicted themselves here.

## 2. Must be a chance of success.

If you were diagnosed with cancer and in one day you could be told your cancer had gone wouldn't you consider that successful? If a treatment can eradicate one tumour in one day most would consider the treatment responsible extremely successful. If a patient had many tumours eradicated I think you would be talking miraculous. Leah had her tumours killed and eradicated by the Gamma Knife. We were over the moon with excitement. She was able to resume work and family life again. Everyone we have spoken to have been amazed by the success of the Gamma Knife treatment. I think the answer to the question posed in criteria 1, above, is that we got Gamma Knife to Australia due to its success and as an option for people who need it. The Gamma Knife was 1000% more effective than any option offered to us in Australia.

## 3. Treatment must prolong life.

Leah returned from Melbourne after having her whole head radiation and there was no change in her condition. Her oncologist was very apologetic but said there was nothing more that could be done. Leah was advised to get her affairs in order. Then after having Gamma Knife she was able to return to normal life again. She saw her son start school, saw her daughter commence high school, she had several more Christmases, birthdays and special occasions. The treatment gave us, not only extra time with Leah but also gave her increased quality of life. The criterion doesn't indicate the definition of how long life must be prolonged. Is it a percentage, number, formula or what? We were offered no scale to compare with. What if they did have a figure, you had treatment and died one day beforehand or one day after that stipulated date? This was such a confusing aspect of our application being denied that even my solicitor couldn't explain it to me.

4. Treatment must be recognized as a genuine treatment.

We were accepted on this criterion as Gamma Knife has been used since 1968 and was in the process of being considered for use in Australia. If it had of been in Australia maybe all of this would not have been needed.

The criteria in the MTOP application were too subjective to offer consistency. We just wanted to help Leah, found a treatment that worked and then a payment option was to be found at a later stage. I think we were well within our rights to access the overseas treatments. In Australia chemotherapy had helped but hadn't cured the cancer. Radiation had almost killed Leah yet made no difference to her health, except in a negative way. Chemo was not even an option at this stage. Yet we sought a treatment, which cured not 1, 2 or 3 tumours but many and was considered by our experts to have failed. After assessing all this information my solicitor was very confident of a favourable result. This was some good news for a change.

I know my emotions come in to it. But even with emotions aside the MTOP funding criteria is very subjective and can vary from one case to another. There are no guidelines or formulas as cancer doesn't allow this. Why is chemotherapy considered effective yet 40,000 Australians die each year whilst this is their main treatment option in Australia? Figures can be deceiving. You are considered a cancer survivor if you last five years after having treatment. If you die one day after that date you are still considered a cancer survivor. It's horrific how figures can be manipulated to suit a purpose. When I received notification that my MTOP application had been denied my heart sank. I cried again. I felt sick and I didn't know what was going to happen. I didn't know how we were going to survive. I didn't know we even had the avenue of an appeal. But we could appeal even though I was worn out both emotionally and physically. It had taken months just to get to this stage. Having the solicitor take over this responsibility was comforting. The banks and now the government had really pushed me as low as I could get. Was I beaten? Would the appeal be successful? Only time would tell.

Some other interesting things happened around this time. One was an article I saw on breast cancer and the spokesperson they were using to promote this cause was famous Australian model Sarah O'Hare who married Rupert Murdoch's son, Lachlan and became Sarah Murdoch. I contacted her when she was hosting The Today Show on Channel nine in Australia. Now Cyberknife was not used to treat breast cancer, as such, at the time. However if a patient got secondary cancer as a result of breast cancer then Cyberknife could play a major role in recovery. I explained about Cyberknife to Sarah and she responded, quite excitedly, a couple of times and then just as suddenly she stopped replying to my correspondences. I sent her videos of Cyberknife successfully treating patients. I sent information which areas within the body Cyberknife can treat. I sent her photographs and patient stories. By this time a number of other Australians had been mentioned in the media as having had Cyberknife overseas as well. As much as I tried I could not get her to show any more interest in this cancer treatment. Her profile, contacts and influence could really have made a difference and we could already have been saving some lives from that time. It was disappointing that she snubbed us but I had been in this situation before so no surprises there. That was when I found an annoying precedent. A friend of mine from the Gold Coast had escorted her friend to Malaysia for her Cyberknife treatment for an inoperable brain tumour. Gold Coast media, The Bulletin, radio and even NBN television, have been very supportive and pro active in many facets of my varied battles so it came as little surprise that they jumped all over this great story of survival. However it did not remain local. The local media informed 60 minutes of Colleen's story. The people at 60 minutes were extremely excited. The producers dealt with Colleen over the phone to get a brief history of the situation. After this initial interest there was lots of hasty communication to ensure that the story went ahead quickly. The producer set everything up. They arranged suitable times and places for the filming to happen. I had been through the same scenario so I could identify with everything Colleen was experiencing. It is exciting but a nervous time as well. Colleen felt the same obligation as I felt about informing people about Cyberknife. Then just as rapidly as all of this had started they stopped contacting Colleen. She endeavored to re instigate the communications but it never happened. The story faded away. Colleen's friend continues her good health today but she could have impacted the choices of so many others had 60 minutes, televised by Channel nine in Australia, gone ahead with the story. A pattern was emerging. Channel nine had now dropped the ball a couple of times in quick succession. This was both very frustrating and disappointing.

All of this was very frustrating but I had my own life to consider as well. I also had a huge commitment to my children. They were doing well but I had a wakeup call at a parent teacher interview. Both the kids had adjusted as best as I could expect after such a traumatic time. However when I met with Rebecca's teachers they showed concern. Her grades had dropped. I queried this and they explained that they had shown Rebecca quite a bit of leniency over the past few months. Being a teenager she had lapped this up. Unfortunately this was a few weeks from the end of the school year. I was disappointed that I hadn't been informed prior to this. But what was done was done. I loved the school. Bec had been involved in numerous activities that we were invited along to. As Leah's death was still quite recent I would become quite emotional at these events. I was so proud of what Bec had achieved and also proud on behalf of Leah who would have loved to have seen these performances and activities. Alas, Leah could not be present and that is why they were such emotional experiences. This was also the reason why I was quite frustrated at the slow reaction of the school with Rebecca's lapse. We discussed this issue at home. We had a bit of a family meeting. I wanted to support the kids but I needed help, as well, from them. It was lovely that the school had gone easy on Bec but they had done it for too long and now Bec had suffered. So it was now time to bring Bec back into reality. We discussed the issue and I gave her a school term to turn her results around. She was a very good student so I knew this would be easy for her to do. We also looked at the children assisting me at home. I had gone pretty easy on her as she needed extra care being the only female in the house. I had encouraged friendships with neighbours who had mums and could chat with her and support her over a cup of tea. I asked for help around the house as when we had bed and breakfast guests it was quite demanding. Bim was a great help and would assist me in looking after the guests we had staying at Leahbelles. However Bec wouldn't pitch in. I am not sure why but she stood firm in convictions not to assist. I explained that I was fine with her not helping but that effort would also be reciprocated by me. I also indicated that I had gone out on a limb to ensure we hadn't been required to move. It was a decision that I had no difficulty making but I could have sold up straight away and saved all this drama with the banks. However I had given her my word that I would try and save us from needing to move. I was disappointed that she showed little support for me with my small requests for help. But I was still aware that she had lost her mum. So I let it ride for a while. Her grades didn't improve so I was forced to change her schools. This was actually a benefit to her as it took her out of her comfort zone and forced her to react. She did react in a positive manner and her grades improved when she started at the local High school. However at home she still refused to help. I am not sure if this was due to the fact that Leah used to do a lot for her when she was younger. But now she was older she needed to take on more responsibility. This, however, did not happen. I would have to deal with this for a while but my main concern was her school work which had improved so I was happy for that. Rebecca was a good kid so I figured the rest would sort itself out.

# Chapter 23

# Got to love the media

Three strikes and you're out. That was my philosophy about some of the media I had dealt with.

Not long after all the Ebay and MTOP fiasco we were in the news again. I was really struggling financially, even more than before. I was going backwards about $1000 a month at this stage. I had a decent cash flow but when I got ahead in one area another needed attention. Fees, charges and penalties, issued by the banks that refused to refinance me, were crippling me. I was watching TV one night and the advertising amazed me. It was about 2am and I had an idea. Not quite sure of the sense of the idea but I was being ignored through mainstream avenues so had to continue looking outside the square. I decided to promote my back as advertising space for any company wishing to use the space to have their logo placed on it in the form of a permanent tattoo. I had quite a list of media contacts so put it out there. The things I felt I was forced to do just to get by. The things I was doing to provide for my kids. I couldn't just sit by and wait for the MTOP or I would lose the lot.

Some of the banks had already threatened to take our house off us. So I sent the information out about offering my back as a billboard. I got inundated again. Responses came from the media, tattoo artists and a few companies wishing to take advantage of my offer. A Current Affair, shown on Channel nine, contacted me and wanted to do a story on me. Oh no, I thought. Here we go again....

They came out and spent the day interviewing me and the children. They then took location shots of our property, the bed and breakfast and our surroundings. They had a sound and camera crew that was flown up for the day and the interviewer and all his equipment. It was quite a draining day. Questions had to be answered in such a manner to be suitable for television. They took photos and video of my auction site for the back, pictures of Leah and other background props that could be used to make the story well rounded and create impact. Then they packed up, gathered their gear and headed off. The story never aired. Channel nine had again pulled the plug, so to speak.

Just as this was happening, a producer from Kerri Anne, a morning show on, yep you guessed it, Channel nine also contacted me. She wanted to know if I'd be willing to have the tattoo done live on the show. I had already arranged a tattooist, numerous clients and now the TV show. I was amazed that this could actually be happening. They were going to fly me down to Sydney to have the tattoo done live on the show. They would pay the air fares and transport to and from the studio. My cousin heard about this and she was disgusted that I had been put into such a position that I had to face doing this sort of thing just to survive. She said that when I was on the show she would ring up the Kerri Ann show and start an auction to stop me from having to get the tattoo. I laughed. I was blessed with great family and friends with such love and caring towards us. I started to prepare for the segment on the show. I had to have the kids looked after. I had to get to the airport. It was a bit to organise but not too much that it was a hassle. The hassle would be living with this tattoo after the show. I had deliberately chosen the back as it could be kept covered. But just as quickly as all the interest had began, the production team stopped communication again. The segment never went ahead. To this day I have not been able to get a response from them. Channel nine had struck again. Our local media heard of all this and came up and did a story for the local Byron Bay newspaper, The Echo. This, again, ended up being more about the Cyberknife than assisting our situation but it was good exposure for one of my causes. The local media had been exceptionally supportive of us in all aspects of our fight. They took a photo and super imposed a tattoo of the "Echo" logo onto my back. They included more of our story and it ran in the paper the following week. Channel nine's lack of support, however, was a setback. It was a setback both in the fight to get exposure for Cyberknife and to help us financially. My 2am brainwave had failed. But at least my appeal to the government regarding my MTOP funding would be resolved soon. Hopefully common sense would prevail and with the funding I would be able to pay off a substantial amount of the cancer debt. If the funding had been granted at the time of application the entire amount would have already been paid back. A number of years down the track and this debt would now only be partially paid off. This had been both wasteful and frustrating. The only winners so far were the banks.

I received a small amount of luck just afterwards though which offset some of the frustration. One of our local radio stations, ZZZ in Lismore, was running a competition. The winner had to have an interesting story and get the most registrations / votes from friends or colleagues. A friend entered me and I was excited by the $3000 prize up for grabs. The radio station rang me to discuss, on air, my story. I had gone through this so many times in so many forums that I almost had it down pat. The DJ who interviewed me was extremely moved and off air wished me the best of luck. My story was deserving of the prize apparently but so were many of the other stories. I crossed my fingers and actually forgot about the competition until I received a call a few weeks later letting me know I'd won. I got the most votes and the girls at the radio station had great delight in ringing me with the good news. I was so excited. I was also a little shocked as not much had gone right for quite some time but I was over the moon with joy. I had to go to the radio station to pick up my cheque. I did this and thanked all the staff who were there to greet me. It couldn't have happened at a better time as I was due for a mortgage payment that day. So I promptly deposited the cheque onto my mortgage. The money was gone in an instant. No treat. No splurge. The windfall just vanished into the black hole that was my debt, my life of the last few years. The sad thing is that it didn't even make a dent in the amount I owed. I was just paying interest. So the minimum that I struggled with each month just kept my debt at the same level. The win was amazing but it also pointed out one poignant thing. A "little" amount such as $3000 didn't achieve anything. I needed a huge injection of funds to make inroads in to this situation. The funding from MTOP would have been such an injection but unfortunately this seemed like a solution that may never be reached. Still, Leah's positive outlook had intervened again. I had kept optimistic throughout this entire chapter of my life. I used to joke, with friends on the phone, about having to hang up because a cheque was in the mail as I spied the postman stopping at our mailbox. This is a positive affirmation technique used by Leah for years. It actually worked on many occasions. I would go to the mail box and there would be a cheque. It was never a life altering amount but a figure like $30. I would laugh but in reality it was enough to buy groceries or petrol for the car. Even this small amount was a bonus and I was thankful for how lucky we were to have received it. Many would have rolled over and given up by now but I still remained positive to try and fulfil my children's wishes of staying in their home. A little win such as the $3000 I just received renewed my optimism and gave me hope that I was heading in the right direction. Leah was a huge advocate of positive affirmations. Well she had to be when faced with her situation over the years she fought cancer. This way of life had rubbed off onto many of Leah's friends as well as myself. Without this positive thinking I don't know where I would have been.

After all my frustration and disappointment with Channel nine over the years, I got a call out of the blue from a journalist at the Gold Coast Bulletin. He had followed our story for a while and wanted to do an update. It sounded good as many people had seen tiny aspects of our story but this was an opportunity to fill in some gaps, go behind the scenes of our lives and put our adventures into some sort of perspective. We made a time to meet and he came down to have a chat. I had done articles before and they were great and usually contained a piece on what I was up to at the time and then a tiny bit on the Cyberknife. This was quite an in depth piece. It started at the beginning of Leah's cancer journey through to the present, at the time. It covered the need to head overseas for treatment, the success of the treatments, the disappointment at the eventual outcome, the frustration of the financial strain we were under and some of the unique ways we had tried to buy some time or even eradicate some or all of the debt. But this article touched on some of the positive events in our lives as well. It came out in the big weekend edition of the paper and took up an entire two pages. The articles heading freaked me out a bit. "What drove us to sell Leah's ashes" was the title. It was created to grab people's attention so that they'd read further. I got a lot of phone calls about the article and people were extremely sympathetic and encouraging. I made some new friends due to the article. People enjoyed the fact that it created an entire story and not just the sensational bits of my life that were used in short bursts as shock value. It created more interest in Cyberknife but in the end it didn't help our financial situation. I was happy though to be able to tell the entire story. Many people read this throughout the Gold Coast and beyond. I ended up helping many others again.

People who read it wanted to access the Cyberknife. I was more than happy to help in any way I could. So, after the article, my life returned to normal. Well what had become normal for me anyway. I don't think I liked normal if that was what I was in the middle of experiencing. But as I had said all along, if I just laid down and gave in to the banks or the Government, I would have been crushed and faded into oblivion. I had to be the squeaky wheel for my own good, for my children and even for complete strangers who deserved better. I had met many new people throughout this process, many who had been complete strangers, who had been so supportive, genuine and generous with time and thoughts. The Gold Coast Bulletin article had put me in touch with many more people who offered support to us or were asking for support themselves. The story in the paper had further raised the profile of Cyberknife in this country as well. Little by little word was getting out about Cyberknife and we were hopeful of a positive outcome to our situation. As Leah used to say about her cancer journey - little baby steps. Our life over the last few years had been just that. Little baby steps to try and keep what we cherished. We had managed to keep our lovely home. We still had our security and our support network. We had chipped away as best we could at this mountainous debt. I remained hopeful.

A great result out of this exposure was that I was contacted by a solicitor and a financial advisor who asked me to come and see them and they'd see if they could help with my refinance situation and assist with my debt consolidation. I had been unsuccessful at getting my debt repackaged so it would be more manageable and now I was excited by the opportunity of some professional assistance. Hopefully they could succeed where I had failed. I brought in all my information and they were confident all could be resolved. They advised me that the main issue was to eradicate all the unsecured debt which was created when we needed quick funds upfront for Leah's treatment. It seemed bizarre to be still talking of this several years after Leah's death. I had thought I could have fixed this up within weeks or months of Leah's death. But now years on I was still paying up to 25% interest on that hefty sum. But these two experts were confident they could help. At this stage I was closer than ever of losing everything so needed all the help I could get. I spent a few months liaising with the two of them and various financial institutions. We applied to many. I got rejected by most. I got to the valuation stage of financing with a couple of lenders. I had about $200,000 equity in the house but that still wasn't enough to get approval. My unsecured debt was the hurdle. It was a catch 22. I was trying to eradicate the unsecured debt by transferring it to my mortgage. By doing this my monthly situation would have been extremely manageable. At a lower interest rate and spread over the life of the loan, the repayments came down to a sensible amount. By this stage the debt from the cancer treatment had almost doubled due to the high interest rates, penalties and the like. Most institutions declined my applications due to the amount of unsecured debt I had. It was frustrating as that was why I was applying. I was trying to eradicate that part of my debt. Another issue during this process only added to my situation. With many of the applications, once initial approval had been granted, a valuation on the property would be ordered. In just a short amount of time, over a couple of years, I had ten valuations done on the property. As they were $600 each I had actually lost another $6000 as these refinances had not gone ahead. It was very frustrating. During this stage of my life I was working three jobs. My current expenses were around $5000 per month which I had shown the ability to pay for nearly four years yet I still couldn't get anything through. Then finally after a huge amount of investigation and effort we found a lender who might be able to help. It was noted and brought to my attention that it was a private lender and not a bank. It was a private lender from the Gold Coast. They would lend the money. But the application fee for it was to be $30,000!!! I kid you not. The interest rate was to be 12%. This was half the rate of interest I was paying for a huge portion of my current debt so it didn't sound as bad as it looked. But the upshot of all of this was that I had a six month contract with them. I would have the 12% rate for only six months. If I made the required payments, for the six months, without problems then I could refinance at the current industry rates which were about 6.5% at the time. Six months of pain to get a good result. The figure of $30,000 really scared me. I felt sick to the stomach again. I had been backed into a corner and this seemed to be the only way out. But after looking at the bigger picture I could see light at the end of the tunnel. I went to the solicitor to seek his advice. He said I had no options. I either sold the house if we could find a buyer. I had made the promise to my kids not to move so I declined this option. It wasn't really an option anyway as buyers were scarce. He said I could default on my current situation and lose the house or take this new refinance option. The one bright light out of all of this is that my credit file, at this stage, was still in good shape and if we could consolidate through this lender, it would remain so. We spoke about the consequences of going ahead with this loan. What if I missed a payment? This would make my credit history a bit shaky and then the next refinance may not proceed. How much would it cost me per month? It would be $4200 which was less than I was paying now but with the $30,000 application fee I would not clear all my high interest debt. So I would still have some other repayments as well. All in all, even though I would be going backwards again with the $30,000 upfront fee, it seemed manageable. At least the six months would go quickly, a new refinance would happen and my life would be back on track. I would be able to budget and plan for the future at long last. My initial feelings of uncertainty and trepidation gave way to excitement for the future. After all, unlike previous borrowing attempts, this deal was guaranteed to go ahead. So I had to pay $30,000 application fee, borrow some more money and pay 12% interest on my mortgage. Was this an offer too good to refuse? I hope you can sense my sarcasm! Why are the most vulnerable the ones that people take advantage of?

We had moved to the Byron Bay area five years before. We had a simple life. It was bliss. Our debt was around $200,000 in total. We were cruising. My debt now was going to be over $400,000. I was terrified. This "solution" also did not clear all my unsecured debt. The $30,000 application fee meant my personal loan with Citibank would be left to deal with still. That was at 19% interest, so still quite expensive. But it was the lowest interest rate of the debt left after paying for the cancer treatment. More new debt to clear the old debt. I just felt like packing it all in and walking away. Wouldn't that be easier? I had been through this before and had decided to stick it out. I had my kids to consider. They were secure here. I tried to shelter them from the harsh realities of the financial situation we were in. But when dad gets off the phone to the bank in tears or a daughter asks for money for female hygiene products and we have to borrow the money from a neighbour, they become aware that all is not as it should be. Every cent I made in the last four years had gone to the banks and yet I had gone backwards. If I had known that the banks were going to be so heartless maybe I would have done things differently. But my logical solution to all this had made sense at the time. The ANZ had even approved my loan several years ago only to back down at the last minute, so I must have been right about the refinance option. If I had known that the government wouldn't pay for Leah's treatment through the MTOP, which is there for such purposes, maybe I would not have pursued this course even after promising the kids we'd be alright. At least it would all be sorted out by me accepting this deal with the private lender. Maybe it was a path I had to take. A roundabout way of getting to a place I thought I should have been years earlier but maybe this new deal would help our lives start to make sense again. Time would tell.

# Chapter 24

# Citibank and yet more media

I was at Bim's soccer training one afternoon. It was
4.59pm. Training was almost over. My mobile phone rang.
It was Citibank. I had been waiting for my new refinance to
settle so I could start making normal repayments again. I
had not paid Citibank for a few months but my solicitor had
rung them weeks ago and asked for a moratorium on my
payments until this had settled. They were hesitant and
obviously now had decided on other measures. They had
rung to say they were defaulting on my personal loan with
them the next day. I had one minute to act. They were so
generous. This was around the time that Citibank had been
bailed out in the USA during the global financial crisis. The
assistance they got was in stark contrast to the assistance
they had offered me over the years. Now they were placing
their boot on my throat and going for the kill. Citibank had
tried to rain on our parade but I was determined not to let
them. The media became a big player in my life again. I
quickly rang my solicitor and explained my predicament. He
was disgusted. He had negotiated my situation with them

and was under the impression Citibank were happy to assist so they would get their money. Obviously this was not the case. Due to my list of media contacts, my solicitor rang Channel seven after Citibank had rung me about the default threat. Today Tonight rang Citibank and said it would be fine if they put my account into default but that they would like to do an interview with them about the situation and the way it had been handled by Citibank. They explained that I had already scheduled the interview with their reporter. They would have a film crew at Gold Coast airport first thing in the morning. This must have scared Citibank a bit. They backed down and then rang to discuss a solution. I was disgusted that it took media intervention to prompt this response rather than any goodwill on their behalf.  ABC radio also rang to cover the story. They did an interview about our ongoing predicament and why the banks and the government had turned their backs on us. We were also in the newspapers again. I think the children were tiring of it all. I know I was. However, as you can probably imagine, I always looked for a positive outcome.

This positive outlook on life has nothing to do with Citibank but my son's soccer team. The Mullumbimby Hornets. Bim loved his soccer and a couple of amazing things happened in 2009. His team was doing well. They had only lost one game. A few weeks after the Citibank fiasco we were all at training and a tragedy unfolded before our eyes. Young Matthew, who was one of the players, was not there. The coach came in and told us the news that Matthew had died. He had been at the game the previous Saturday but fell ill later that night, was rushed to hospital but died on the Sunday. A lung infection of some description. We were all totally inconsolable as you could well imagine. He was such a lovely young boy. Now he was gone. The club had organised a counselor to help the other children. They did activities. They wrote cards for Matthew's memorial and signed Matthews guernsey which would be placed in the casket at his funeral and then retired. I couldn't fathom any of this entire situation. With all we had been through this was just another shocking experience. I couldn't imagine what Matthew's parents must have felt at that time. I had lost a partner which is horrific but to lose a child would be devastating. Bim was really upset as he and Matthew looked after each other on the field. They hadn't known each other before soccer but had grown close due to soccer. This was one of the hardest experiences I had encountered. I had to comfort Bim during another life altering situation. A bad situation, again, unfortunately. Being a bit older I had experienced several deaths, including Leah's and my mother's. But this was so unexpected. It took us all by surprise. Bim was visibly upset. The entire community was changed by young Matthew's death. It felt very unfair. It is a terribly difficult memory to write about. But it doesn't end there. The Hornets made it to the Grand Final. The final was held on a beautiful morning, a few months later, in Byron Bay. The coach met us all and told us we were playing the Grand Final in Matthew's memory. He was dedicating it to Matthew. We hadn't won it but how could we be denied? He told the players that they'd be wearing black arm bands. We had to explain what that meant. We had to help the kids wrap the black tape around there arms. Well, all the parents were beside themselves. This was to be an extremely emotional day. The kids won. Bim played a blinder but all the others did to. It was like they were not going to give in until they'd won. Which they did. Then they had the presentation. The soccer federation had made a set of medallions for Matthew and they were presented to Matthew's parents. Oh my God. With all the excitement of the win and then this we all broke down. But it was an honest display of how we all felt for young Matthew and his parents. They must have been so overcome by the emotion displayed by the players, coaches, parents and supporters. This was a huge day that would live in our memories for ever. A few weeks later we had the presentation evening. The Hornets had worn light blue guernseys throughout the season. They had won the premiership for Matthew and the club announced that they would never use the light blue guernseys again. All the guernseys would be retired in Matthews honour. He had been part of the journey, he had played that year. He had passed away and the team went on to win. Mullumbimby is a tiny town (the biggest little town in Australia, so the sign says) but they sure know how to support, honour and  celebrate someone special. Matthew's parents took part in presenting the trophies to the players and they all got their light blue guernsey to take home forever. Bim never played soccer again for Mullumbimby. He wanted to the following year but with our financial situation we decided the money could be better spent elsewhere. The banks needed it. To see Bim put our family first was amazingly admirable. But it broke my heart. The club actually offered to pay for Bim's registration and insurance but he was a bit embarrassed so we declined the generous offer. Our time with Mullumbimby soccer was special in many ways. Leah had gone to the early games and got so excited by all the action and how well Bim played. Not that she was biased!  My cousins, who had visited at one stage, came to a game one morning and loved the community feel. I enjoyed the social aspect and diversion from my woes and would get caught up in the excitement of the games. Bec would come down and bring the dog and get some fresh air. It was a very special time for us all.

Now I had to deal with keeping our heads above water. I had been naive, in hindsight, to believe I would obtain approval from my bank to refinance my financial situation upon our return from Oklahoma. I had held on to the hope that my government would allow me funding, which everyone I spoke to, thought we were eligible for. I had placed Leah's ashes on Ebay after being backed into a corner. This created a huge response but nothing tangible that I could use to rectify our situation. I had offered my back for a tattoo of a company's logo but it never eventuated. I really couldn't see a way out of all of this. I was losing faith and patience. But I had delayed Citibank's intention to default against my loan. My new mortgage was soon to be finalised. I still held out hope.

Then the journalist from our region's major newspaper approached me again. He had seen the recent situations I had been confronted with and he wanted to help. He had met Leah and knew of our hope with the Cyberknife treatment a few years prior. He could not envisage, at the time, what we were going through now. He was aware of the events that had impacted on us during that time. His paper had even covered some of them. He wanted to become involved once more. He invited me to come to the opening of a film mentoring program which was being launched the next day at a community hall in Bangalow. The mentoring program was being funded by the federal government and our local MP, Justine Elliott, would be there to preside over the proceedings. I didn't understand how a mentoring program opening could assist me but he assured me that getting the minister involved couldn't hurt. I agreed. I could have a chat to her and see if she could assist in any way with getting our health minister to look at our situation compassionately or if there were any other avenues in which we could proceed. I turned up to the opening and the media was everywhere. This must have been a bigger announcement than I had first thought. This mentoring program must have been quite significant to attract all these media personalities. But I was wrong. They weren't there for the opening of the program. They were there to ambush Justine Elliott and force her in to acting to come up with a resolution for our dire situation. I sat and watched the speeches and official presentations for the opening of the mentoring program. It was quite interesting. Then Justine made her speech. Then she left the hall and was immediately confronted by television cameras and journalists. They initially asked a few questions about the program she had just opened. Then they switched the focus to me. I had written to Justine before so she knew of my story. The journalists asked me to explain it anyway so the viewers or readers could get some background. Then they asked Justine what she could do to help. She covered it all up by saying she couldn't say anything due to confidentiality laws. I said I was happy for my private details to be aired. My God I had had aired my soul on national TV, radio and news off and on for a few years now. But we had to buckle and Justine and I went off to the side to talk privately, while the cameras still rolled. She had agreed to take the issue up with the federal health minister, Nicola Roxon. This was a start. After all an election was looming. I had to make them all understand that we had gone overseas as we had been given no options in Australia. The treatment had worked. If the government had a fund for exactly this purpose surely we were entitled to utilise it. That was all I could get across. It's all I thought I needed to get across. Surely the evidence would speak for itself.  A few weeks later Justine's office rang to say they had sent a letter off to Nicola Roxon. They were sending a copy off for my reference. I got this in the mail a few days later. I should have guessed things were not looking promising after the envelope I received was empty. I rang Justine's office and mentioned this and a filled envelope was sent to replace the empty one. What and who was I dealing with? Incompetence on a huge scale. Did Nicola Roxon also receive an empty envelope? Why was cancer such a difficult thing to make any progress with? Why are our government representatives so hard to communicate with?


A month or so later I received the standard letter from Nicola Roxon's office stating that no funding would be forthcoming due to the fact that Leah's treatment was not successful. I still could not fathom how a treatment that cures numerous brain tumours can be deemed unsuccessful. This battle was set to continue. All avenues had been exhausted, explained Ms Roxon. That was that.

# Chapter 25

# A win in West Australia, a loss at home

I had a number of people from Perth in West Australia contact me about Cyberknife. I had not thought too much about Perth as I knew little about it. I figured the East Coast was the place for Cyberknife to get introduced to Australia due to its ease of access and population. People could fly or drive or catch a bus to access Cyberknife in a city such as Sydney or Melbourne. Well in India, they have two hospitals offering Cyberknife. Patients ride their bikes to the hospital to get treatment, have the treatment and then ride home. Amazing.

My new friends in Perth suggested petitioning the West Australian government. They had lots of spare cash due to the mining boom. What a great idea. If Perth got Cyberknife we may not be able to ride our bike to access it but we could get a cheap flight, catch a train or bus or get a friend to drive to Perth. We began to look at this option seriously. I even got people to join in and help. I started another

Facebook page - "Let's make West Australia the first state in Australia to get Cyberknife". It had all the contact details for the Premier and the Health Minister. More information on Cyberknife and its benefits as well as videos and photos. It got great support right away and still does well today. Little did I know the impact this would have on the direction of Australian cancer treatment for the future.

On the home front it was still a struggle. Financially anyway. My Bed and Breakfast was doing well. I had a good job at a TAFE college and I was coping alright with the huge expenditure required of me each month. The children were coping well. Rebecca still didn't want to help around the house but friends assured me this was just a phase. All teenagers were like that. It was frustrating but I just had to monitor the situation. I had spoken to her a while ago about consequences. She was learning about these with her attitude. She was at the age where some pocket money would come in handy. In my day I helped out to earn pocket money. She didn't like this idea. I can't understand why she didn't want to help. Surely the money wasn't the only incentive. But I wasn't able to hand out money just for the sake of it. But not having pocket money meant that she missed out on things due to her stubbornness. She came home one day and said she wanted to get a part time job after school. I thought this was a fantastic idea. Maybe the structure and social nature of a job would help her in other areas. We put together a resume and she approached the local deli. She got the job. It meant that I had to get up at 5.30am to get her to work by 6.00am for her to open up the shop, prepare the display and get ready for the first customers. I wanted to support her as best I could so this was not a chore. If I had Bed and Breakfast guests I was up early anyway to cook the guests breakfast. So Rebecca began work, was still doing well at school and I hoped she would regain her old enthusiasm once more. Around this time I got more bad news. The college I was working at did not get enough enrolments to employ me with the usual hours I had been getting. They could only offer me two hours per week. My, oh my, what was I to do? This left me way short of the amount I needed each month to cover the mortgage, let alone living expenses. This was yet another hurdle I would have to deal with. I would need to last about six months on this reduced income, until a new semester, with new students, came about. I didn't know if I could last. I had to look at my options. I rang the real estate agents again to see what the likelihood was of a quick sale. They were not overly optimistic. These were still uncertain financial times we were experiencing. I asked them to begin getting things together anyway as it was now quite urgent. I know I had promised many people, my children included, that we would be able to keep the house but it was becoming increasingly obvious that this would not be the case. I had run out of energy, funds and ideas. I had promised the children but I was now being faced with the fact that the government was determined not to help us. The banks had turned their backs on us and forced me into a shady deal with private lenders. Things were not good at all. I was disgusted. Now I had a new deal with a lender which I may not be able to honour due to the reduction of working hours and therefore income. My little plan to use this deal in the short term, to allow for a longer term solution, was starting to fall apart. It was the thing I feared when I first looked at the new mortgage but I figured six months would fly by. I had only one option. Sell the house. I thought I'd take matters into my own hands to speed up the prospect of a sale. We had three alpacas that were used as lawnmowers to keep the grass down. They were gentler on the property due to the padded feet. We had run horses on the land before to keep the grass short but they dug up the ground with their hooves. The alpacas were also a unique aspect for the Bed and Breakfast guests. I thought I could utilise the alpacas to my advantage at this stage of proceedings. The real estate market was flat. Our home was a lifestyle property rather than a practical residential house so the interest was slow. Decisions of this nature were not rushed. I was in a hurry though. So I advertised the alpacas for sale, with a free house thrown in. It got in the news again. From Lismore up to Brisbane. I had quite a bit of interest. But as I would need at least $500,000 for the alpacas, this interest soon diminished. After all they were not show or breeding alpacas but mere lawn mowers. This hadn't worked and I now had to look at other alternatives. Quickly. During all of this I was having a chat with a friend one night not long after and I joked about walking away from the house and the debt, giving the house away so the banks couldn't get their greedy little hands on it. I had tried unsuccessfully to go through all the logical channels available to me. I had done some fairly bizarre things as well and fallen short. Maybe walking away was the best option. We had a station wagon and could sleep in that for a time.  Then, as we talked more about the situation, walking away and moving on, other options sprung up. Not the most mainstream but options just the same. The most logical, in a funny sort of way, was a raffle. The more we thought of this, the more achievable it seemed. What if I was to sell tickets at $100 each and we got 5000 buyers? This would cover my debt and give me a few dollars left over to start afresh. Someone gets a house for $100. No agents, no bank phone calls every day. A deadline of say 30 days. My troubles could be over. Except we'd be homeless and my promise to the kids would be broken. Well this is how my life had been for some time now. At least I would not need to default on the loan so I would be able to rent or indeed, in the future, borrow again for a new home. I would do it. I spoke with the children about it. I had promised Rebecca during the week of Leah's funeral that I would try everything to allow us to keep our home but that this was not going to be possible. It's not like she was showing any concern for her home anymore. I think she had lost interest. She was actually okay about it all. But both the kids had gone without so much for so long. I think Bec had endured enough. She had control over her little nest of security that she had set up and now that was getting taken away. I sensed she changed during this time. She wanted out.  Bim was very casual about things, like myself, and was happy to go with the flow. So a raffle we would have. I searched for information on running a raffle and discovered I would need to apply for permits in each state that the raffle would run and, of course pay a fee. This was going to take time and money, both of which I was seriously running out of. Then I saw another option, not a raffle but a competition with a task to be achieved by applicants. Because no element of chance was involved in this sort of thing I didn't need to apply for the gambling permits. This would be quicker, cheaper and the added bonus of being able to promote something as the task that people had to perform. I decided that the task each person would have to perform was to create an information page on the internet explaining Cyberknife as a cancer treatment. I made a Facebook page called "A house near Byron bay for $100". It still exists. Still has nearly 1000 "fans". I then promoted this page to my ever growing list of contacts to see what the reaction would be. Well it went berserk. I was woken at 6am the morning after my email by a Sydney newspaper. They wanted to run a story on my competition. So a photographer was sent up to take photo's and gather some information. The next day a big story featured in the paper. I was a bit disappointed by the lack of response but one little story created a snowball effect of reaction. Firstly Steve Liebman, who is a fairly well known journalist in Australia, rang me to interview me on his radio show. He rang mid morning and we had a chat on air about most of the stuff you have read about in this book. He was very sympathetic and hoped I would get a reaction from the politicians involved in the refusal of our funding for Leah's cancer treatment. The other result was that from that interview I was again inundated by enquiries about the Cyberknife and how people could access it. The next day I was again rudely awakened at 6am by the media. The newspaper story and the radio interview had sparked a bit of curiosity. Our local paper in Lismore also ran a story on the front page. Our little idea was growing quite significantly and maybe we could pay our debts off after all. The first phone call that morning was from Channel seven. They wanted me to appear on their evening current affairs program. I had done it before so I had no hesitation in agreeing. They had been very supportive of me over the years and had played a big part in saving a number of lives due to people obtaining Cyberknife treatment after seeing the first story they ran on Leah's journey a few years before. I then got a phone call from Channel nine. They wanted to do the story also. But they wanted me to reject Channel seven's advances so they could have exclusivity. I was not impressed by Channel nine's treatment of me over the years and their attitude toward helping cancer sufferers so I politely declined. Channel seven got the story. Channel nine wanted to show the story on A Current Affair, which may have had more weight but I would stick to my guns and allow Channel seven to run it. The show aired and a friend rang me after seeing it. While I was talking to her I could hear the beeps on the phone indicating other incoming calls. This was constant. When I hung up it was a continuous stream of calls from people wanting to purchase tickets, wanting information and various other enquiries. I sold about one thousand tickets in a few hours. The number of Cyberknife information pages began to appear immediately. Most of these were on Facebook. That was fine. It was all information and publicity for numerous causes. Some Facebook pages had fans by the dozens by the end of the night. I then got another call from the Sunrise morning show which is also aired on Channel seven. They wanted to interview me live the next morning on their show. I had already received about one thousand enquiries about the competition in one day as well as numerous queries about getting Cyberknife for cancer patients. Complete strangers rang or emailed to pass on their thoughts, prayers and well wishes. It was all quite overwhelming and gaining momentum. I had to go to Ballina racecourse early the next morning to be part of a live cross from the studios of Channel seven in Sydney. The presenters on Sunrise wanted a chat with me. Everyone was quite taken by my ingenuity and guts. But really I had been given no choice over the past few years but to come up with bizarre means of survival or the only other option was to roll over and lose everything. So the Sunrise story created more of a stir and more applications to take advantage of the $100 house. I had to reach 5000 applicants or the competition would not go ahead and I would refund the money. I got a lot of fans on the Facebook page but a lot just wanted to offer support and couldn't or weren't able to offer the money to actually take part. The information pages for Cyberknife were quite imaginative and many in numbers.

Some of the titles for these pages included:

Cyberknife miracles

Cyberknife for Australia. PM Mr Rudd have a heart (this was changed to Ms Gillard after the election later that year....)

Help bring Cyberknife to Australia

Cyberknife - Australia needs you

Cyberknife - Why is Australia 5 years behind?

Cyberknife where the bloody hell are you?

and many others.


A website was also created by one of the participants which was phenomenal.

www.cyberknifeaustralia.com

This had a wealth of information, stories, contacts, links, case studies and information on our plight. It was professionally done and had links to Facebook and twitter and had interactive forums and blogs. I even got contacted at this time by a doctor from Florida in USA. He worked with Cyberknife and heard about our plight. He actually offered me, or actually Australia, his services and that of his team of specialists in the use of Cyberknife. They would come over and train Australian staff in the use of Cyberknife so it could begin use as soon as we got a facility. We are still waiting. I wrote to the West Australian government and offered them this great opportunity. I got a response which I should have expected. They were pleased with the offer but declined the gesture. They assured me they could staff a centre on their own. You have to laugh. If you took it all too seriously you'd do yourself an injury. Then just after this response we got some fantastic news. All the petitioning of various governments had paid off. The West Australian government had responded quite favourably over a period of a year or so. Many people from the support site sent letters to the West Australian Premier and Health Minister. They had received very positive responses. We actually got quite personal responses rather than the generic responses we had gotten from many other government departments. Then we got confirmation that the government in West Australia was actually building a new cancer facility at the Sir Charles Gardiner hospital and that they were including a facility for a Cyberknife. Unfortunately the centre wasn't to open until 2012 but it was a start. Hard work does pay off. But one machine for 20 million people is hardly sufficient, so we will keep persisting. They didn't have Cyberknife in the UK either a few years ago. But constant petitioning over there resulted in the first Cyberknife being installed a while ago. Now they have several. So it looks like once an initial system is installed others want it as well. That's the way we had to look at it for Australia anyway.

Some other people contacted me, due to the exposure of the raffle and offered to win the house but wanted the children and I to stay and live there. A few wanted to win it and for me to stay and run the bed and breakfast. Others just offered to buy the property, which I couldn't accept at that stage because I had committed to the competition. It was an extremely hectic time. I endeavoured to reply to everyone who contacted me. It all took time. But people had been so generous. Some contacts were via the mail. I had some people who would monitor the site, on my behalf, if I was busy at work or with other commitments. I was very lucky to have these people in my life. I couldn't have done it without them. The competition had a one month deadline. The first week had been phenomenal. It would remain to be seen if the rest of the month continued the same. By the end of the month I had nearly four thousand people get behind me, support me, show compassion and about one thousand, five hundred actually paid $100 for a ticket to help me out and possibly win our home. But unfortunately by the cutoff date we did not have enough applicants for the contest to proceed. So I had to inform people of this sad fact and begin the process of refunding the money. Organising the refunds took over a month as I had to cross check each deposit with the name of the person who submitted it and then go to my bank account and initiate a transfer back to the persons account. Some of the payments were done on Paypal, who thought the popularity of the account activity was of an unusual manner, so they decided to freeze my account. I then had to offer the refunds out of my bank account, which never really has the most substantial balance in it anyway, as you've probably already discovered!

The other thing with Paypal is that they charge fees. So the competition actually cost me quite a bit. But I had to try something. I had to look for another positive out of this bizarre venture. The good outcome was that I was able to utilize the funds temporarily deposited into my account to keep things ticking over and keep the banks at bay. I was still working, the B&B was doing well and by the end of this whole process everyone was paid and I was still afloat. Just.

The whole episode took a few months and my hours began to increase at the college so things were manageable again at that time. We had a number of people come and visit. Some about the house. Others about the Cyberknife. Some then ventured off overseas for treatment. I made many new contacts throughout this time. People interested in real estate. People who wanted to help more with the cancer treatment even though the competition had ended. People who were going to go overseas to access the treatment either with or without government help. I met couples with young children needing something like Cyberknife as no options could be offered in Australia. I met politicians and media people and the support all around was amazing. It was like a little network with everyone trying to help each other in some way. My thinking at this stage then began to change. I was now moving in a new direction due to the fact that I was able to face up to the reality that we might have to move. I had faced fear many times in the last few years. I was fearful of letting people down but had to push that to the side. I had no options any more. The banks wouldn't help. The government refused to help. My options were gone. I had fought off bankruptcy but still faced losing the house. I was over it. My kids needed to move on. We all did. I was sick of paying off huge amounts each week or month and getting nowhere, going backward even. With the rate of interest I was paying I actually looked at the reality that over the last few years, even though I was somehow able to keep making my mortgage repayments, I had paid nothing off. I had paid over $100,000 but I was still at the same place, financially, I had been for four years. I hated the fact that with all the interest, fees, charges and penalties I had just given away so much money. Money I could ill afford to lose. Money taken away from my kids. My future was becoming more apparent to me. The fact that I had been open with the children and now other family and friends, the possibility of a move was becoming a reality. Really I had been holding on to the house for the wrong reasons. I was doing it for others. Even though I had amazing memories of the place. Leah's monument was built there. A beautiful magnolia was planted in her memory. It was thriving. It never flowered while we were there. It had buds on it as we were about to leave. This was a sad realisation. But I also took solace in the fact that it was just a house. Bricks and mortar (or weatherboard as was the case here). Our memories would go with us. We had hundreds of photos. Hours of video. So many stories of this time and many others. This was going to be okay. I also wanted to leave with good memories of Leah's final place of residence and not become too bitter about the time spent there. I wanted the good memories to outweigh the bad. I wanted this phase of our family's time to be remembered for what it was, the pain was part of that but we had many beautiful and emotional memories as well. Both with Leah and also since her passing. These were the things I wanted to take with us. I didn't want to develop any feelings or memories based on a financial situation that was generally out of my control. So this is what we would do. The process, both physically and emotionally, to move on, had begun.

# Chapter 26

# On a personal note

Now for a story of something totally unexpected that happened in my life at this time. It was rather life changing but in this instance it was a change in life I was only too willing to embrace. This occurred during my time conducting the house "raffle". To promote the Cyberknife and also highlight the unfairness of not having it in Australia, I would contact politicians via email, letters or on Facebook. Facebook was good because I could attach photo's, video, petitions and things of similar value which others could see and place a bit of pressure on the recipient to act. One NSW politician was Barbara Perry. There was no particular reason I contacted her but fate played a role here. She responded a few times, we actually added each other as friends on Facebook, but it must have gotten a bit "political" for her so she deleted me and stopped replying. However one time when searching for her on Facebook to send a message I clicked on the wrong photo. But the message was sent anyway, not knowing it was to the wrong person. I got a harsh response from the recipient a day or two later. Who are you? What do you want? What's all this cancer stuff? Her name was Karen.

She was from Sydney. She was a friend of Barbara's and had been to school with her. I replied to Karen with my deepest apologies. However she responded again. This time she replied in a more receptive manner. It turned out that her father was not well with cancer and she was actually interested in knowing more about the treatment. I responded again and after she looked at my Facebook profile and the Cyberknife information, she told me she remembered me from the television segment I'd done a few years earlier on Channel seven. She had watched it with her mum. She had turned to her mum and commented on how upset she was for my family and I due to the death of Leah and our financial strain. The tone in her correspondence with me changed. It became caring and sympathetic. I felt for Karen and the predicament her father was in. I had met so many people searching for options in the treatment of their cancer. Karen and I communicated quite regularly after that. The correspondence with Karen actually became more frequent and more personal. By New Year 2009 we were actually dating? But we'd never met. Michael Buble released a song - Still haven't met you yet. It was uncanny that this was released at this time. This was exactly how our lives were unfolding. We talked over the phone about Sleepless in Seattle. A love story about a widower who falls for someone he has never met. We rang each other several times a day. I bought a nice writing pad and I wrote letters and scented them with my best aftershave. I was enjoying this attention and the ability to reciprocate. I hadn't had the opportunity or allowed myself to be like this for years. I had been for coffee with girls that may have had the potential to lead to more but I didn't have the inclination. I didn't feel I was in the right space and I felt it wasn't appropriate to feel such things. Not that I was actually feeling such things previously. I was beginning to now, though. I think it was fortunate that this was a slow progression and we had the distance between us. This allowed things to move along slowly but gradually. Sydney to the North Coast wasn't just an impulse trip. Since our initial contact and after some research of her own Karen became a strong campaigner for Cyberknife. Then she did a really brave thing. On the weekend of Valentine's Day 2010 (yes another milestone happening on February 14th!) Karen took the gutsy step of getting on a plane and flying to Gold Coast airport to visit me. She had arranged it then informed me. I was amazed. Karen flew up in the morning on the Saturday. I picked her up at the airport. We went for coffee to see if there was any spark first. She stayed at my Bed and Breakfast for the weekend. We were hooked. I was amazed that I could have these feelings again. I had just assumed I would spend the rest of my life alone. We really enjoyed the weekend just getting to know each other. I was able to leave the trials and tribulations of my life on hold for a few days. We talked, ate some lovely food, walked, sipped wine and coffee and just enjoyed each other. She wanted to know about Leah. My life had been on show but Karen was getting to know the man behind the story. It was bliss. The two days flew by and soon the weekend had to end. Karen had to board her flight and return to Sydney. I felt different after that weekend. Anything was possible.

The next week I rang Karen's mum to assure her that my intentions were honourable. Her mum sounded nice. We had a brief chat and Karen was impressed at my ingenuity in obtaining her mums number as I only had Karen's mobile number. She was flattered by my decision to ring her mum. Her mum had joked that Karen was foolish flying up on a whim as I may have been a lunatic. But after my phone call Karen's mum and dad must have talked. Karen's dad gave her the money to come up again a few weeks later for another weekend. She came up and met my children. They had been at a neighbours the time before that Karen had visited. That meeting all seemed to go alright. I did not know how the kids would react. I think they were happy to see me happy for a change. They were wonderful in accepting Karen and being so welcoming. It was also so generous for Karen's dad to pay for her to visit. I would later find out that Karen's dad was a very generous and delightful man.

A month or so later Karen arranged a trip to the Gold Coast for our combined families to get to know each other. She had booked a beautiful apartment in Broadbeach. It would be good for Rebecca to have a few female influences for a change. I thought the time away would be good for her. Karen brought her daughter with her who was about a year younger than Rebecca. We visited a theme park while we were there. This was such a treat for all of us. This was a fun day which took our minds off the bad things that had happened in our lives and we were able to enjoy some fun. Then we did some shopping at one of the huge shopping centres on the Gold Coast. I couldn't remember the last time we had done that. We cooked and had barbecues in the lovely apartment we had for the week. Karen took Rebecca clothes shopping and had her fitted for a bra. I didn't even know you could do that! This was nice experience for Rebecca. She was able to do the personal things a girl needs without the embarrassment of having dad around. It was a rare treat for Bec. Karen made a declaration to me at that time. She said to me that she could never, nor did she want to, take Leah's place. It was a genuine sentiment and an honest comment. It was touching. But we both had children already and we needed to be there for all. This had started nicely. It was working well. This was a wonderful opportunity to experience something quite different for all of us for a while. It was not all smooth sailing but life generally isn't anyway. The distance would be an issue but neither of us was in a huge hurry if it meant rushing things and causing ripples. We were able to enjoy our time away before our lives would resume as normal. Sure enough after the wonderful holiday it was back to our respective homes and back to normal. I did go down to Sydney to meet up with Karen again for a weekend. I still had frequent flier points from years before. I decided to use them. We toured around Sydney and its many tourist highlights. I knew very little about the city so it was a great break. Karen also took me to meet her parents. I had spoken to her mum previously on the telephone but to meet them was amazing. Her father was so welcoming, warm and generous. He couldn't do enough for me. Her mum is a gem. She is such a natural and warm hearted lady. They were both full of life and wisdom. It was my pleasure to meet them both. It was a short meeting but extremely enjoyable. I liked my time in Sydney with my new love. I did miss my kids though so it was nice to return to them. Karen and I had seen each other's worlds and we liked them both. We would make this work. We were now used to the long distant relationship with the odd catch up in between. Things were going along nicely. Unfortunately a few months later Karen's father passed away from his illness with cancer. This was such an unfair situation. Not that cancer is ever fair. The only positive out of that whole awful time was that I had the privilege to actually meet Karen's father. It would remain a strong memory in my life. The world had lost another kind, generous and loving man. A father, husband and valued member of his community. He left a huge gap in so many lives. My life was also the poorer as a result of his passing. I was blessed to have met him though. Karen's family has such great stories about him and at least I can say I met him. It allows me to picture him in these lovely family memories.

Karen has shown support for me even with all my previous issues. It was touching. For the first time in a long time I was Ash. She didn't look at me as the poor guy who lost his wife or Leah's husband who is doing such a tough job of looking after her or whatever other description I had been given in the past few years. It felt nice to be a person again. So we are still going along nicely. Karen helped me with the raffle situation but in the end we had to move from the Byron region anyway. However for the first time since Leah's death I look forward to the future with positivity, enthusiasm and hope.

# Chapter 27

# In the news again

Life was still moving on. It wasn't ideal but I was still making progress. I was approached to do a television interview regarding a class action being organised against the banks for charging unjust fees. The people organising this had seen my story, followed it and thought I could be a good example of the banks exploiting their position and taking advantage of people held to ransom by them. I had paid thousands in fees over the last few years. I wanted to fix the situation but the banks had declined. I had closed all my accounts but they still charged me fees each month. I tried to reason with them over the years but it all fell on deaf ears. They had refused all my attempts to rectify my situation. But I figured it made sense for the banks. This was easy money for them. They were reaping hundreds each month for doing nothing. Why change that and make things easy for me and then miss out on high interest and high charges? I was forced to toe the line or I was charged even more. Others were probably in similar situations but as I had been in the media quite a bit the group organising the class action figured I would be the perfect example to highlight the action on the television news that night. I agreed to do the story. It was a chance for me to get one back against the banks. It was a bit ironic that the first bank they were seeking judgment against was the ANZ. My bank. The bank I had been with for years. The bank I did all my business banking with. The bank that had approved my refinance years ago, which could have solved all my problems, but then turned their back on us. Channel seven was doing the story. The cameraman came to my work while I was on a break and we went to a local park and filmed it. They just asked what types of fees I had been paying and I answered. Yearly membership fees even though I had closed the accounts and was not able to use them. Late payment fees, overdue fees, over limit fees. It was also about how the fees were added to maximise the impact for the bank. After the interview had finished that afternoon the case was lodged with the Federal court against the ANZ. I still have one outstanding debt with them today which I am slowly reducing. This was a test case and if successful the group would follow other banks in pursuit of justice. The next bank they would instigate proceedings against was to be Citibank. Wonderful. The two least compassionate banks were top of my list and also top of this groups list. I would be actively involved in that case also. I had paid thousands over the years and apparently it only costs the bank a few dollars each time any of these fees are added. The process seems to be a huge profit making exercise, hence the class action. It remains to be seen what the outcome will be but I can only hope for a few dollars out of yet another ordeal. At least with this episode other people are controlling the progress. I just had to sit and wait. However I am not holding my breath as I have been tantalised before with the offer of a refinance and the MTOP application, only to be disappointed in the end. Still it's worth a try. Nothing ventured, nothing gained.

After the raffle had ended I had to make some huge decisions. I hadn't raised the money needed to pay out my loans. I didn't have sufficient income to pay the monthly amounts of my current mortgage and the residual high interest debt. I shrugged my shoulders and admitted defeat. It was heartbreaking. I couldn't go on. It was time to make the move. Rebecca was almost at the end of her year 11 studies so this would be as opportune a time as any to move to our next place. Both emotionally but also physically. I got the real estate agents in and I signed up. I had to sell quickly. I would take the first or quickest offer. They had said that it was their responsibility to try and get the best price for me that they could. I didn't have time for that. Just sell it and get whatever they could and as quickly as they could. My mortgage was now costing me $6000 a month. My contract had expired with the lenders initial generous offer of 12% interest on my mortgage and now I needed to pay default interest. It was 18%. I couldn't do it. I contacted them and explained that the house was on the market and I was selling dirt cheap. I needed a sale at any cost. The figure I put on our home was about $200,000 less than market value. That should create some interest. The figure was roughly the same as what I would have gotten if the raffle had been successful. However as this was months later I had paid out nearly $20,000 in interest in that short time. Wasted money as it was just paying the principal and not reducing my debt. This had to stop. We got interest in the property straight away. We conducted many open houses. Several a week to ensure people were able to come and see it and be tempted. Then I got an offer. I accepted. Things began to happen. The move began. We had to find a property to move to. The Central Coast of NSW was the desired destination. This was a seemingly nice region but had the added advantage of having more infrastructure than where we were presently. Things were closer. We would have more choices. I was getting emails from Central Coast real estate agents with rental properties available. We found one. We liked it. It was suburban but with a National Park opposite. It was close to the beach and a lovely lookout. So it still had a sense of space. This would be our new home. I now needed to start packing. This took quite a while and many memories came flooding back. It was comforting. It was cathartic. It was difficult. It was refreshing. I could feel the burden lifting from my shoulders with each piece I packed. We would be taking these memories with us not leaving them behind. We would need to leave a few things but it was a sacrifice we had to make. The beautiful magnolia tree which marked Leah's memorial. It was too big and established to remove and then relocate. I cried when I visited this spot for the last time. I weeded around the base. I could feel a presence. I was saying goodbye again. This was difficult. But the tree would remain. I would be able to see it from the road. We would revisit from time to time. We had friends in the area still so it would be nice to come back. Another thing that was hard to leave was a mosaic that Leah had created. Years before we had even met Leah had visited a fortune teller. She had told Leah a number of things that had come true. I was one. Bim was another. Travel. A country property. And cows. Black and white cows. We used to laugh about this. Even when we moved to the country we had no intention of getting cows. The milk would have been nice but getting up early to get the milk and the upkeep of cows was off putting. But Leah had worked on a mosaic with her friend Jacinta when we moved to the house. It was a landscape. Our landscape. When it was finished I fixed this to an exterior wall of our renovation. It was on a deck so we'd sit by it most days. It was magnificent. It featured cows. Black and white cows. We laughed. It was the final prediction the fortune teller had mentioned. It had been unexpected and unintentional. But Leah had her black and white cows. We couldn't take that with us as it was fixed to the wall and was now a fixture. It would remain at Leah's final residence. I thought it was fitting. Sad but fitting.

While all this was happening one of my contacts sent me an opportunity of sorts. It was a link to a website for the

Victorian government at the time. It was asking for ideas from the public of ways the government could improve things for Victorians. I replied and suggested becoming the first state in Australia to offer Cyberknife. Even though this would be in Victoria it could benefit all Australians. It could create medical tourism opportunities, it could increase cancer care choices for Australians. I sent this suggestion off and more of less forgot about it with all that was going on at the time. A few months later I read an article in the Melbourne newspaper about a study tour to Japan by representatives of the Victorian government, the media and experts from the Peter Macallum cancer hospital in Melbourne. They toured the many hospitals in Japan offering Cyberknife. After this study tour, the Premier of Victoria promised $8 million for the Peter Macallum hospital to establish Australia's first Cyberknife centre. I got phone calls of congratulations from many people far and wide. We had won. This was great news. The Victorian government issued a press release and substantial advertising indicating the progressive measures they were taking to make Victoria great. One of the points stated that Victoria was to become the first state in Australia to have a Cyberknife centre. However a few months later there was an election. The government was beaten. The promise of Cyberknife was withdrawn by the new government as a cost cutting exercise. We were all so disappointed. We had made such progress, got the response so many had wanted and it was all gone again. Just another frustrating episode in my life recently. This was a small distraction during the time of our move. It had been exciting and even though it ended poorly I realised we were heading in the right direction.

Around this time I also had a small discipline problem with Rebecca. I can hardly blame her. I could only imagine the emotional and psychological pressure she must have been under. She was obviously frustrated by the predicament she had created. It was fine not helping out around the house. But with that came the consequences. I was busy and didn't have the time to do certain things for her. A lift to the movies was out of the question if she was not willing to do small tasks for me. It was a stance I needed to take for her future. But it certainly made her a bit more imaginative in the way she could obtain things. I was still working, which included a couple of nights at the college, so I asked Rebecca's grandparents for help at this time as Rebecca had misbehaved quite mildly. It may have been a small incident but it could have had dire consequences if things had gone poorly in her little plan. She had put herself in possible danger and deceived me. It was very unlike her. However I felt she needed to be disciplined. I could have made her computer off limits but with me working a few nights she would just get on it while I was away. Her grandparents lived on the Gold Coast and I asked if Rebecca could stay with them for a few days to be supervised as I couldn't while I was at work. I explained, even if briefly as not to alarm them too much, what Bec had done. I let them know that this was a punishment as well. They agreed to help which was a relief. They were retired and still found it so hard to believe Leah was gone so this would be a way to keep their minds off things while helping me out. They loved to spoil Bec as well. They had always been like that. But this was for discipline not a treat so I made sure they were aware of that. So I sent Rebecca up to her Grandparents for a few days after we had quite a serious conversation about things. I explained the punishment and the disappointment in her behaviour. The fact that I was scared for her safety. I had explained to her numerous times in the past about consequences. The next few days would allow her to reflect on these. I still had to work at night that week so I asked if our neighbour could look after Bim. She agreed and all was set. On the Thursday, a few days later, I went up to the Gold Coast to pick up Bec and bring her home. I hoped that the time away had made her realise the consequences of her actions. She had only been away for a few days but we both missed her. When I arrived at Leah's parents home

Bec wasn't there. I asked of her whereabouts and was informed that they had put her in school on the Gold Coast. Well you could have knocked me down with a feather. I really didn't need this at this stage. We discussed the situation but they felt it best for Rebecca if she stayed with them for a while. They had already enrolled her in school so how long was a while? I tried to work out what was happening but couldn't actually do anything as Bec was at her new school. Queensland has a different system to NSW so it was going to be very disruptive. I don't think they had thought this through very well. A solution wasn't going to be arrived at that day so I said I would come up on the weekend to sort it all out. I talked about the possibility of Rebecca having some counseling. Running away wasn't the solution. We had to deal with this situation. She would get some spoiling at her grandparents but I don't think a reward for misbehaving was appropriate. It may have been nice for Bec but not the right course of action. I know the last few years after her mum's death must have been really difficult for her. As it was for all of us. But with Bec's age and needs it must have been harder for her. She had created a bit of a safe haven at home and maybe a short stay with Leah's parents would be just the tonic she needed. I hoped so and would find out in a few days. I had to leave the Gold Coast as I had Bim at a neighbours. But I went home on my own. Just another time I had to deal with the unforeseen on my own. I also had to explain Bec's absence to Bim. But I told him that he could come to pick her up on the weekend. Sunday was Father's Day and we would go up, have some lunch with the kids grandparents and come home as a family again. This is what we did. We went up and Bec was a bit sheepish. We had lunch, had a chat and then I asked if Bec needed a hand with her things. But Rebecca had been thinking about it and she wanted to stay. I was shocked but didn't want to force the issue. The time after lunch became a bit awkward. I don't know what pressure Leah's parents had put on Bec but she was adamant that she was staying. Nothing I could say or do could persuade her. This was ironic because the kids used to be amazed at how patient I was with Leah's parents because they frustrated them. Don't get me wrong. They loved them but found them difficult unless it was in small doses. I was very patient with them as I felt Leah would want me to be. I never gave it a second thought. But I was becoming a bit frustrated with them now. However they are very persuasive people and it was obvious Bec wasn't coming home today. After lunch Bim and I left. By ourselves. On Father's Day. The drive was about one hour. It was silent for most part. I had to explain to Bim what was going on but aside from that it was quiet. I was mulling it all over in my mind. I had battled with the banks in the hope that we could stay, till this time, in our home. I had made a conscious effort, a promise, to do this so Rebecca could finish year 11 and not be too disrupted and then she could start year 12 in a new school. She would now still be in year 11 in Queensland schooling for another term. But I wanted her to be happy and safe. I don't know about happy but she would be safe at her grandparents. I had done everything I could for Rebecca. I tried to keep the house as she had asked me to do during the week of Leah's death. I had tried so hard to fulfill her wishes but the harsh reality of the real world, in which we live, had taken over. I had gotten up at 5.30am to drive her to her part time job. I had driven her to early school classes. I had gone easy on her input around the house. She had it pretty easy really. But she also missed out on quite a bit. Throughout her entire life, from when she was just one, I had done the best I could at the time. I thought I had done alright. I had asked about teenage girls with friends and neighbours and they'd had assured me that all was well with how we were going. But I was feeling really hurt now. However if Rebecca was safe that was the main thing. I had lost my wife a few years ago and now I was losing a daughter. I had lost the most important role I could have. That of a dad. This had been taken away from me without consultation. To make matters worse I still faced the reality though that we still had to be out of our house. Maybe after the 2010 school year was over Bec would come home. To our new home on the

Central Coast. Only time would tell. I now had more hurt and more pain to deal with. I hoped it would end soon. Enough was enough. A lovely correspondence I received at this time came from a friend. It was just a simple message.

*"Promise to my child - I will hound you, freak out on you, lecture you, drive you crazy, be your worst nightmare, until one day you understand why. Because...I LOVE YOU."*

I only had a few weeks left at our home. I would ring Bec and see if she had changed her mind. We went up again to visit. She was staying. It was gut retching for both Bim and I. A few days later the removalist arrived and we were gone. We had a three day trip to the Central Coast which I was looking forward to. Three days without banks, in laws, media or a house!!!! The only thing I could influence at the moment was our future. I had to get Bim settled in his new school. I had to set up a house and had to try and get Bec to come to her senses. We moved in October. It cost a lot to do. The house sale was progressing but very slowly. As I had no savings it was a difficult time financially. But this was not new to me. Once the house settled I would have a little bit left over which would help for a while. But I now had no job. We were in a new region and it was like starting from scratch. It was actually quite refreshing. This was the feeling I had when we moved to Hamilton Island. A sense of liberation. It was also the feeling I had when we moved to the Byron Bay region. We knew nobody. Had no jobs. But things work out. There is that transitional stage where things sometimes go a bit pear shaped but generally we adapt and progress.

The government had rejected my funding for Leah's overseas treatment which forced my hand. Forced me into selling up and moving on. They may have saved a few dollars by denying my claim but now I was back on welfare. I hated it. But gee I was lucky to have it. I had gone from being a property owner with two jobs and a business to needing government assistance again. It had a negative impact on me as well. Over the years I had been successful in many areas of my life. Finances had always been strong. We had travelled extensively. I had completed numerous areas of training and personal development. I had wonderful employment opportunities and much responsibility. I had always been a jovial, relaxed but professional person. I had a wonderful family that I was and still am proud of. But the last number of years had been horrendous. You can only take a certain number of knock backs. I think, if it weren't for the number of successes in that time, the end result may have been different. I had become a shell of the person that I once was. It would take some time to get back to somewhere like that man again. Could our new life in a new area provide the spark that I needed? How long before I would find out? It wasn't long at all. I found work in a sandwich shop. Not the most glamorous career choice for a 47 year old man but it would pay the rent and allow me to meet people and contemplate my future. It allowed us to settle into life on the coast well. But one thing struck me. I had paid tax all my life. Thousands of dollars. I had owned properties and businesses. I had been a teacher. A mentor to some. I had helped people get lifesaving cancer treatment. I had been around the world trying to save my own wife. My kids mum. I thought I was quite grown up. I had done the right thing. Then when I needed assistance from the government they rejected my appeal. So here I was. Nearly 50 years of age. I was working part time making sandwiches. I was renting. I had no savings. I felt like I was 15 again.

# Chapter 28

# Sold

Our house at Wilsons Creek finally sold. We were moving on with our lives. Not that we were leaving the past. We would bring the important parts of that with us. We had hours of video and dozens of photo albums. We moved to the Central Coast of NSW and waited for settlement of the sale of our house. Of course this dragged on and on. As I was paying $6000 a month on my mortgage at the time it cost me a fortune while we waited for settlement. It took nearly three months. Another $20,000 wasted. Then the lender I was with, Strone Properties, demanded over $10,000 in exit fees. Added to this were the legal fees of several thousand and so on and so forth. So I came out of the sale still owing a bit but it was over. I had a few odds and ends to clear up, which would still take a few years to finalise but the experience with the banks was over. I was in no hurry to enter in to a mortgage again. Renting was just fine at that time of our lives. I now had to concentrate on replacing lost time and experiences with my family and friends. I still feel ill when I think of the wasted four years my kids had to endure waiting for something to happen, that never did. I set up a savings account and actually put some money aside each week. It felt strange but secure. Security was something we hadn't experienced for years. What did the future hold? I wasn't sure. We had been forced out of our home. I lost a good paying job due to the move. I lost my daughter and placed myself into the public eye with sometimes humiliating results. So the future had to be better than those last few years. Don't get me wrong. I had lived in paradise with Leah, initially, and our two brilliant children. I made some lifelong friends and had some wonderful experiences but faced a lot of adversity and hurt as well. I was quite unknown on the Central Coast so it was a chance at a new beginning. I was in the news so often up North that I faced public scrutiny quite regularly. Not that I minded at the time. If I could help people I was happy. If there was the chance of rectifying our financial situation it would have been worth it. One consolation is that I was able to avoid bankruptcy. I came close a few times but just managed to keep my head above water. That's only money though and family, love and friendship is far more important. With the benefit of hindsight I may have done things differently. If I had known now what I needed to know then maybe our present would be quite different. But you can only do what you know at the time. My first thought was for the children. I needed to look after them after their mum's death. I thought I was doing the right thing. As I have said the logical solutions to our problems appeared so easy to attain. In the end neither came to fruition. So we had to leave that part of our past behind. Rebecca eventually left Leah's parents care on the Gold Coast and moved in with her God parents in Melbourne. She completed her HSC year 12 at Leah's old school. Maybe she needed to find herself. She may have needed to step out of her comfort zone and look towards the future. It hurts so much to have tried so hard to help her, quite often at the detriment of Bim, but that's just one of life's little hurdles. We will work on it and hopefully a happy solution will eventuate. I have to thank my cousin, Cheryl, for her help and supportive words during this time with Bec. She has raised two kids and had similar experiences raising them, so she was able to offer some guidance and support for me when Rebecca left. Cheryl's kids are adults now but are great people so I look forward positively. It's these little experiences that I take a great deal of comfort in. My little efforts to help others sometimes seem insignificant but when I hear positive results I realise the impact they can have. My life has been filled with similar offers of assistance and they have been gratefully accepted and appreciated. Rebecca will not be left on her own. She has a lot of support from family and friends. She is progressing well and will do well at university. She won an art award for her major work during her HSC. She was featured in the Melbourne newspaper as a result. We were all so proud. She is studying nursing at university which makes me happy. Some of the nursing staff we met throughout Leah's journey were inspirational. They work long hours in difficult circumstances but have an amazing impact on the people they are helping. Rebecca will make a brilliant nurse.

This was where my initial attempt at writing this book ended. I had no money and no assistance in putting it out but I did it anyway. I have since had a number of amazing experiences with the book and was asked to update it and release it locally. I will continue our story from that point on now.

As I said I worked in a sandwich shop when we first moved to the Central Coast and I must thank the owners who took a big risk employing a 47 year old single dad whereas they normally hired 16 year old kids. They had never hired a male before either. After the interview the owners asked the other staff their thoughts on hiring a guy. The other staff said at the time that women are better at multi tasking and they were all a tad apprehensive about employing me. However one of the females suggested that men can concentrate on and do one task better though so I should be given a try. I am still looking for that one task that I can do well. Not sure what it is. But being the first male employed by this shop was a milestone and I was there for many months so it seemed to go alright. I wanted to get in to teaching again and there was a lot more opportunity on the Central Coast with colleges, community schools, private training companies and the like. I also looked at doing a Leahbelles type business again but that would have to wait.

Speaking of Leahbelles. I wrote a letter of thanks to all the guests who had stayed with us over the years and the responses I got were quite amazing and very emotional. Some of the people had new babies, some had lost partners and others wanted to catch up for a visit in the future. Most had been saddened by the need for us to sell up. And some actually said they had tears as they read my letter. That's the type of experience Leahbelles was. I put my heart and soul into it and I think the guests felt that. I wanted to endeavour to keep in touch with these guests who came as customers and left as friends.

Bim did so well with the move. He ended up being very happy in his new school. He moved from a school of 50 students to one with 700. It was a big change for him. But he jumped at the opportunity. He could do things we weren't able to previously. He even formed a band and produced a two track cd, a dvd and performed a live concert. He was still only 11 years old. He had enjoyed playing guitar and got very good. He didn't play soccer when we moved but he played Aussie rules football. He had never done it before but became one of the better players. The coaches loved him and he won a regional award for his efforts. Bim made a number of new friends in different areas of his life. School, footy and music. It was a good mix. Bim also nominated me for father of the year that first year. My goodness how could he? He had gone without so much. He had lost so much. How could I even be considered for an honour such as that? The story was featured in our local papers. This included a photo of the 2 of us. The entire community fell in love with him. The sandwich shop I worked at actually laminated the story and put it up behind the counter. The customers at the shop loved the story. They also liked my maturity. They could chat to me about stuff the youngsters weren't knowledgeable of or weren't interested in. Life at the sandwich shop was good for me socially as well. It paid the rent and was an outing for me also. The story in the paper obviously embarrassed Bim hugely. But I was humbled by the nomination and proud of my little boy.

As for me? I had a new love. She took a huge risk with a guy who nearly lost it all. At the time in life we were at we should have been thinking about a future optimistically with much more security but we felt like a couple of young kids just starting out. No money, no house but respect for each other and a wealth of knowledge and experiences. Travel had featured in both of our lives and we wanted more. I envisaged travel due to the desired effect of this book. I wanted to travel to promote the book and its purpose to create better options in cancer care for Australians who needed it. We needed to generate substantial donations and awareness to get the Cyberknife to Australia. As was the case in the UK, once you have one others follow. I also wanted to patch things up with Rebecca. That looked like taking a while.  Who knows? But the future was mine again and the banks or the government or cancer wouldn't be able to dictate which direction my life was to take. I had wrestled control back.

Helen Keller wrote - **"What we have once enjoyed we can never lose. All that we love deeply becomes a part of us."**

# Chapter 29

# Would you like fries with that?

Life had started to fall into place on the Central Coast. The sandwich shop had been a great opportunity for me. I made some new friends and regained some confidence. As you can imagine I had been shattered to lose everything I had worked so hard for. This new lifestyle on the Central Coast enabled me to gradually regain some confidence and dignity. The sandwich shop had started that process. It wasn't my dream job but it was important at the time. The flexibility of hours allowed me to be there for Bim with his transition to a new school. We could walk to his school together in the mornings. I could pick him up in the afternoons quite a lot. He would ride his bike over to the shopping centre in the afternoons if I was working. I was able to take him to his football training during the week and catch his game on a Saturday. The money wasn't great but it paid the bills. These bills were still expensive but were considerably lower than what I had struggled with in the previous years. We were able to explore the new environment in which we now lived. I had excitement in my life again. I was a lot more relaxed living here. Money wasn't the focus of my life any more. It was still a necessity but I didn't have to focus on it every day of the week. Not having phone calls from the banks was a nice change as well.

After Bim had settled in to school he started to enjoy his new environment as well. He gradually made new friends and as he is such a nice boy he was invited over by his new friends' parents. This was nice for him and he quickly made the most of his new environment. He became a very good student at school and won numerous awards.

We kept in touch with our old friends via the telephone, Facebook, Skype, email and visits. As was the case with our home near Byron Bay, this area was a region people liked to visit. So we had visitors from time to time which was nice. I sent Bim up to visit our old neighbours from Wilsons Creek a few times. He could fly with Virgin as an unaccompanied minor. Jetstar didn't offer this service. I guess there were no surprises in that. Our old neighbours loved having Bim for a few days and he loved going back and catching up with his old school friends.

Karen was still living in Sydney as she had her job and family there. She would come up for weekends which was nice. As she knew the Central Coast she was able to show us around and help us discover the area. Karen ended up getting a job 1 day a week in the shopping centre where I worked making sandwiches. She worked for the optometrist there. This allowed her to stay longer each time. Our goal was for her to move up permanently but that would have to wait until the time was right. The Central Coast was also a new audience for my ongoing quest to get Cyberknife to Australia. I had met several people who had tried to access Cyberknife and some more that had never heard of it but wanted to assist. I made the TV news as they heard my story and wanted to interview me about my book and Cyberknife. As a result of all this I got nominated for a small business award. I laughed out loud when this happened as I didn't generate any money. I wasn't really a business but with my support sites and the book I qualified for a nomination. The selectors liked the way I had persisted and managed to get the message out about Cyberknife even when confronted with my own personal struggles. I didn't win the award but in an ironic twist Booktopia, who stock my book, won the category I was entered into. This was also a nice change of direction for the attention I had received over the years. So many of my experiences had been negative and my time on the Central Coast had already brought many positive experiences.

I then got a job with a disability support company. The company negotiated employment for people needing assistance and then I would support these new employees in their role. This company had just begun a partnership with McDonald's family restaurants on the Central Coast. McDonalds would employ people with disabilities and my role would be to assist these people in the workplace and help the managers and staff at McDonalds to ensure this was as successful as possible. I had progressed from making sandwiches to working at Maccas! But it was permanent, it was full time and it was more money. The company I had begun working for was a not for profit so the wage wasn't fantastic but it was good to be on a regular income again. Along with the wage came other benefits such as superannuation, sick pay, annual leave and the like. I had really begun to turn a corner now. I could plan even more. It would still take quite a while to eradicate the debt I was still carrying but it was definitely manageable now. The McDonalds stores on the Central Coast were all owned by the one family. They were very enthusiastic about the ongoing relationship with the company I was working for. They were also the top franchisee in all of Asia Pacific. I guess that's why they had accepted the responsibility of working with people with disabilities so well. They also got to the finals of the National Disability Awards due to the work we were doing and they came runner up to Telstra. The owner went down to Canberra for the presentation and the Prime Minister was handing out the awards. We made the news with this which was good exposure. I was probably on the lowest wage I had been on for years but I was happy. I realised that money wasn't the most important thing in my life. The fact that I was making a difference with these wonderful employees was reward in itself.

The Cyberknife was still a big project of mine. I now had a new audience. This audience was very interested in this technology. I was amazed at how little was known of this revolutionary treatment in regions where it, and perhaps I, had not been in the news. I was driving past a hotel one afternoon and I heard the local radio station was broadcasting from the beer garden. I had a copy of my book with me in the car so I decided to pay them a visit. In between songs the disc jockeys were just roaming around interacting with the crowd. Ugly Phil was one of the personalities there that day. Ugly Phil was a well known radio DJ who was known Australia wide. He had been on Sydney commercial radio for years. He had been in a relationship years ago with Jackie O, who featured in my story previously. They were the "It" couple of Australian radio for a long time. That relationship ended both personally and professionally and Ugly Phil moved on. He had recently taken on the role as drive time DJ for our Central Coast radio station, Star FM. The breakfast DJ's Mandy and Wilko were there at the hotel as well. I introduced myself and explained what I had been doing as far as Cyberknife was concerned. I gave them a copy of my book to give away on air. They also wanted to interview me. Mandy was quite well known for her promotion of cancer charities on the Central Coast. She had numerous friends who were battling cancer. She was enthusiastic about the prospects of Cyberknife. Ugly Phil and Mandy interviewed me and were blown away by our story. They were also amazed at the fact that with all their involvement with cancer fundraising that they had never heard of Cyberknife. I told them I was not surprised as the people running most cancer charities are only looking at research or education and not really looking outside the box in ways to assist cancer patients. Both of these personalities were so supportive of what I was doing that they gave me quite a lengthy time for the interview. It had immediate impact. They got people to phone up if they wanted to win a copy of my book. They asked me to hang around in the beer garden while they conducted the competition. While I waited, people who had heard the interview on the radio drove by the hotel to come and visit me. We exchanged stories and people desperate for help with their cancer or a family members or a friend's cancer came for information and help. One lucky caller won the book and an ongoing relationship was forged between Star FM and me.

# Chapter 30

# Central Coast TV

The exposure had begun on the Central Coast. At Wilsons Creek I got a lot of interest locally and from the Gold Coast. Now on the Central Coast I was getting interest locally as well as in Sydney. The interest was now in the Cyberknife, our story and this book. After my recent radio success the local TV station, NBN, contacted me to ask if I would be interested in doing an interview. It was a silly question. Of course I'd be interested. However NBN is a subsidiary of Channel nine. I had not had any success with Channel nine in the past so did not get too excited about this interview request. However Emma the presenter rang me, confirmed details and the interview was scheduled. I was asked to meet Emma at the NBN studios not far from home. I had organized some t shirts promoting my cause recently so I wore one of them and grabbed a copy of my book. I took Bim along as well. I thought he'd enjoy the experience.

The t shirts I had arranged to be printed were used to raise awareness of various aspects of my battle over the years. They were for sale and a number of people had purchased them. The messages on the t shirts were: "I helped bring Cyberknife to Australia" This had a picture of a Cyberknife machine on it with the slogan. As Oprah had featured in our story I had shirts with the message: "Oprah and I are changing cancer care in Australia". This then had the website I had set up underneath. People could wear this and create the impression Oprah and the wearer of the shirt had helped bring Cyberknife to Australia. Others who featured in this story were also mentioned on the shirts. I had: "Kyle, Jackie O and I are changing cancer care in Australia". I also created: "Kerri Anne and I are changing cancer care in Australia". The irony of this one was that Kerri Anne Kennelly has since been diagnosed with breast cancer. She is doing well in her battle though which is great. The website where people could buy these shirts is:

http://www.cyberknifeforaustralia.com/


So I arrived at the TV station with my Cyberknife T shirt and a copy of my book. I was met at reception and then they escorted me up to a lovely boardroom where the interview would take place. Emma met me and she was accompanied by a camera man. They set up a microphone, some lights and a reflector and the interview went ahead. Emma asked about the early days of Leah's fight. She asked me about the discovery of Cyberknife and information about what made Cyberknife so special. Then she asked about the book. I explained the reason for writing it, the assistance writing the book gave me with coping with all we'd been through and how people at the time could purchase it. I really enjoyed the experience. It was well organized, quick and thorough. Many of my other media experiences had not covered all the aspects of our journey so I was happy that our new beginning on the Central Coast had allowed me to relay to people the whole story. Emma and the cameraman were both blown away by it all. They were amazed with what we had been through but equally amazed by what Cyberknife was capable of and the fact that it wasn't available in Australia. They hoped this story would change things. So did I.

At the time of the TV interview this book was only available online from the USA. It was only available in hardcopy paperback which took a while to get delivered. In this day and age this was not the most effective way to go about selling a book but with no funds available it was the only way I could do it. However the story on NBN created a spike in sales and developed a renewed interest in my book and Cyberknife as a cancer treatment. Things had begun to progress again. The interview was part of the reason I was asked to re write this book and re-release it.

# Chapter 31

# ABC

Things had started to gain momentum on the Central
Coast. After the NBN story word started to get around
about this guy and the cancer treatment. ABC radio on the
Central Coast broadcast from a shopping centre called
Erina Fair. They heard about me and my book and wanted
to interview me. I had been on ABC radio several times
before. I had been on the ABC radio at the Gold Coast,
Lismore, Darwin and Sydney. This had been syndicated
and people had heard my interviews in Port Macquarie,
Coffs Harbour and even Tasmania. Many people had
followed the links on the internet to listen to my interviews.
Transcripts are still available for people to read on the ABC
sites on the internet. The ABC had been very pro active in
their support of me, the Cyberknife and my book. They had
actually assisted people gain access to information on

Cyberknife. They had been responsible for saving numerous lives as people obtained Cyberknife after hearing about it on the ABC.

So the Central Coast ABC invited me to their studios in Erina for an interview. I had trouble finding the studio at first as you enter it through the ABC retail shop in the shopping centre. When I eventually did find it I was welcomed so warmly. As has been the case most times I am interviewed, the staff new nothing about Cyberknife. I spoke to the producer who was in an office next to the studio and she took all my contact details for the future. Then I was ushered into the studio and the interview began. Again I was asked to begin at the beginning. They were amazed of our story. They were blown away by the potential of Cyberknife and they were excited about the book. Then we participated in something I hadn't been involved in before as far as cancer information was concerned. My only experience had been on the Kyle and Jackie O show. I hadn't enjoyed that. I was hoping this would be better. Listeners were invited to phone in. This was quite a shock for me. I was extremely nervous about this as it was such a new experience. We had callers who had loved ones with cancer. A couple of local health workers rang in and said we already had world class cancer care in Australia. They mentioned some of the equipment we already had in Australia. But I argued, due to firsthand experience, that these had limitations and Cyberknife could fill in the gap for many. This was a common response when asked about Cyberknife. Many people got defensive about criticism of Australia's position in cancer care. I think we are led to believe we are a world leader which is a bit misguided. I think we are leaders in research for sure. But as far as treatment is concerned we lag severely behind. Cyberknife could change that. Many of the listeners agreed and even the presenter put forward a case for Cyberknife.

Unfortunately my book was only available online through Lulu, Amazon and a few smaller sellers. People wanted to pop down to the shopping centre and pick up a copy. But they couldn't. The listeners of the ABC were often older people who weren't overly familiar with online ordering or E books. The radio interview had created quite a bit of interest though which was good.

Just after the radio interview ABC television contacted me. They wanted to know if I was interested in a television interview centered on our debt resulting from the cost of getting Cyberknife overseas. As I was involved in the class action against the banks the producer had heard of our predicament. She rang me to discuss our story and then arranged a time for them to come up and film a story. The cameraman, sound specialist and the interviewer came up early one morning. Even though the story was about the debt they were just as interested in the Cyberknife and my book. They were able to work both of these things in to the story. This was for a ten minute story on the 7.30 program and it took the most of the day to film. Some was filmed at home with the lights in a formal interview setting. Some was filmed in the kitchen in quite a casual setting and we even went to the beach and took some outside shots. The interviewer asked to take a copy of my book with him to read. We all enjoyed the day and it was quite productive. The story would air on television later that week. Of course when it did air we got a big reaction again. I got phone calls and emails and interest in all of the topics covered in the segment was stimulated yet again. I was hoping that all this new interest in the many aspects of my life would lead to a solution. This would remain to be seen. I had to be patient again.

The Sydney Morning Herald also ran a story on the debt aspect of my life. They had heard some of the tales floating around and did some investigation into my situation. They then rang me and asked if they could run a story. I agreed and we did the interview over the phone. The journalist was totally blown away with disbelief. He couldn't believe how positive and upbeat I was. But if I didn't maintain this optimism then I feel I wouldn't have survived. The story ran in the weekend edition of the paper but also ran in the Melbourne Age and every syndicated local newspaper in the country as well.

I got a solicitor who contacted me as a result of this recent bout of exposure. He had dug up some history about my situation. He was also involved in the class action against the ANZ bank. He suggested that I should contact the federal government ombudsman and make an appeal against the decision given to me by the Department of Health and Ageing regarding my MTOP submission. I didn't even know there was a Federal government Ombudsman. He suggested that I should have been advised of this option at the time I had asked Nicola Roxon via my local MP at the time several years ago. But I was told at the time that I had no more options. I had joked at the time that I received and empty envelope from Nicola Roxon that I was dealing with incompetence. This new development backed up my theory somewhat.

So I found the contact details of the Ombudsman. I sent off a detailed explanation of my situation. I attached evidence and also contact details. Within a few days I received a call from the office of the Ombudsman. The lady I spoke with was totally in awe of the courage I had displayed in going through what we had been through. However she couldn't help me. Too much time had elapsed since my application for MTOP funding. They have a time limit on such cases. If I had been made aware of this option earlier then they may have been able to assist me. We were even talking about changing law as the decision makers on the panel deciding who gets funding was unfairly assembled. Representatives from countries actually using the technology funding was being sought for needed to be made available. Presently the panel is only made up of Australian and New Zealand experts. However this didn't help me and was for a lot bigger players than myself to determine, if indeed it ever was.

We spoke for quite some time. The spokesperson from the Ombudsman's office was exceptionally helpful. Upon conclusion she did suggest that, if I felt I had been discriminated against due to poor administration, then I could submit a claim for defective administration. This was called a CDDA submission. I searched for the link to forms and started filling them in. I needed the submission details so I contacted Tanya Plibersek to ask for these. I still have not heard back so it is frustrating again. It is a year of election though so with my media contacts we may be able to create some action with this claim.

I have been in this situation before with little result but I can only hope. The other thing that frustrates me is the other claims within the community that get paid out with apparent ease. Throughout my ordeal I have witnessed a young girl who had already had a liver transplant, resumed a drug addiction and was then funded for her trip to Singapore for another liver transplant. I know how her family felt so held no malice toward her but was angry at the people in government who were making such inconsistent decisions.

Not long after this the breast implant company, PIP, were in the news as they had made sub standard breast implants which were in danger of leaking into the body. The recipients of these implants were being offered funding to have the implants removed. Mixed feelings again. Of course I would never wish harm on anybody but these women had undergone this procedure voluntarily and were being funded to have the procedures rectified. Leah hadn't asked for cancer yet when we tried to help her with a world recognised treatment we were denied assistance. So I think as the years have gone on I have gathered a lot of support and evidence to hopefully have a win in the end. We will see.

# Chapter 32

# My book and the cancer council

I was back in the news again. However the exposure these days was a lot more positive. I was able to focus on the future without the distractions of the urgency of my previous financial situation. This was refreshing as any exposure these days was very well received whereas in the past I quite often got mixed reactions. Any exposure I got these days was a lot more positive in the eyes of those close to me as well. I had actually been recognised in the community. I was nominated for a Telstra business award, I got a letter from the Pride of Australia awards and was nominated locally for a father of the year award. I saw these humbling events as a great new direction for me and my family. The other positive news I received, in an ironic sense, was that cancer council contacted me. They had obviously seen the exposure I was getting and wanted a piece of the action. They had seen my book in the news and noted that I was using the funds from sales to go towards purchasing Cyberknife for an Australian hospital. They wanted to know if I would be willing to donate the money to them. I initially thought this was a great idea. The issue I had encountered with raising money was that I wasn't a registered charity. As a single dad I hadn't had the funds to start a trust or foundation so couldn't do big fundraisers until I was more established. I also thought setting up yet another cancer charity as a waste. Australia has about 200 cancer charities, funds, foundations and trusts. Did we need another? All of these had needed to develop resources, get staff or volunteers and create marketing opportunities. We seemed to be wasting a lot of money, time and resources in replicating the same thing over and over. I noted that cancer charities were great employers. Thousands of Aussies worked for these organisations, which was amazing. However there were a lot of wasted resources as well. So much money was wasted in administration, marketing, capital costs and other expenses. These 200 charities were all generating substantial but not really useful amounts in their own right. I had written to many of these organisations years ago and suggested combining funds and resources. There is a lot of pride and ego involved so this never happened. What if the Prostate cancer foundation got together with the Prostate cancer institute and the state Prostate cancer groups? It seemed logical to me that each of these groups could form under the one umbrella and better utilise resources and fundraising.

So the cancer council contacted me and told me they had heard about my book and the fact that I was donating proceeds to assisting with getting Cyberknife to Australia. They asked me if I had considered donating the money to them. I responded excitedly as I assumed they were considering getting behind the idea of bringing Cyberknife to Australia. I asked the lady if this was the case. She informed me that cancer council don't fund equipment just research and awareness. But they'd take my money. I laughed. I explained that many people were already aware of cancer. Not many were aware of Cyberknife. She didn't like my attitude. She explained to me that it was cancer council's policy to only fund research and awareness. I suggested this could change if there was the possibility of saving many lives. She wouldn't budge. So obviously I declined the offer to donate my book proceeds to cancer council. I have had a few similar situations. I will do my own thing until something definite comes up. I wish that we were able to set up Cyberknife as a research project. Maybe we could access some of the research dollars made available for cancer drugs. Cyberknife could be used in trials for willing patients to participate in. I think we could get hundreds, if not thousands, to participate. We have to change or at least be broader in our thinking regarding cancer treatments now and into the future.

# Chapter 33

# Channel Seven (again)

I knew it would happen. I got a phone call from a journalist with Channel seven television in Melbourne. She had just recently lost her father to cancer. She heard about Cyberknife and was angry. Why was this not available in Australia? Why wasn't her father told about this? Why wasn't this technology known of in Australia? She wanted answers and also wanted to create change. She needed my help. I was only too willing to assist. The other thing that had happened around this time in Melbourne was a young girl named Kahlia Wilson was forced to travel to India to access Cyberknife for her cancer. This story had made the newspapers in Melbourne and created a bit of a stir. Research into Cyberknife brought up my details and now Channel seven wanted to do a story. The producer of the program rang me to discuss the details. They would fly crew up as well as the journalist, Karen, from Melbourne. It was to be done at our home so I wouldn't be put out. I arranged to have the day off work and the day was booked in.

Several cars pulled into the drive that morning. Cameras, lights and sound equipment were unloaded. The crew consisted of a cameraman, lighting and sound technicians. The producer was there and Karen the journalist. This was the biggest production I had been a part of. They were doing a big story. It was going to take more than a day to fit all this in.

The story of Kahlia Wilson was to accompany my story. The past and the present would hopefully impact on the future. They would film us that week and then Kahlia required a follow up visit to India and they would tag along for that. They filmed me and asked questions about life before cancer. They also enquired about life with cancer and what was on offer in Australia. They then went on to ask about Cyberknife, how it worked and why I was so determined to get it to Australia. They looked at my book and asked about what I was doing to raise awareness and money to get the Cyberknife to Australia. Then they wanted some location shots. As we were near the beach we went down and did some arty shots of long reflective walks on the beach. They wanted to create some atmosphere for the story. They had to highlight my loss of Leah. Then when Bim came home from school they wanted a shot of both of us walking up a hill. This was actually harder than the times when we had been filmed at our house at Wilsons Creek. We were surrounded by Leah's presence then but now we had to really think back in time to another place. It was difficult emotionally for both of us. The Channel seven guys were very compassionate and understanding. They were professional and empathetic. If we were struggling they paused. They weren't in a hurry. They wanted a quality piece in the end. This was a totally different experience for all of us. The Channel seven people were amazed that they'd never heard of Cyberknife. They were frustrated and embarrassed that Australia was so far behind. They were shattered for this young girl Kahlia and her family. It wasn't fair that she was forced all the way to India to get the only treatment suitable for her at that moment. They wanted this story to make a difference.

The producer and the interviewer left at the end of the day. The cameraman and the sound guy returned during the week to film some more footage. We went up to a local lookout for some more atmosphere shots. They filmed me at my desk at home using the computer to show Cyberknife information I was supplying to people. They showed footage of my book. In the end there was hours of filming done for a 15 minute story. The amount of editing needed would be a huge task for them. The last piece needed for this story was for the crew to accompany Kahlia on her quest to get Cyberknife again in India.

Several weeks later I got a phone call from the producer of the story from Channel seven. Kahlia had passed away. She never got the chance to get to India for her life saving Cyberknife treatment. If it had been anywhere in Australia her family could have made it to any city to get this treatment. To get to India was much more difficult and expensive. They had been delayed due to raising funds for the trip. They got close but the delays had cost Kahlia her life. The family was devastated. The Channel seven producer had contacted me and she told me that the crew were extremely upset. I was shattered. I had never met Kahlia but I got to know her through this story. The newspapers in Melbourne ran stories on her passing. Young Kahlia had worked her way into many strangers' hearts and they were hearing the sad news of her death. More people were hearing of Cyberknife as a result. The story for television was only partially complete. It wouldn't air until they could find another patient willing to share their Cyberknife journey with Channel seven. How many more people needed to die until we got the changes in Australia?

How many more families were to be torn apart by cancer before we got change?

# Chapter 34

# Success in the West

I have mentioned earlier about the suggestion that the West Australian government be approached about getting Cyberknife to a hospital in Perth. I had done this with encouraging responses from them. I had contacted them several times and received very generous responses each time. It was extremely encouraging and appeared to be inching closer to success. I had created the Facebook group – Let's make West Australia the 1st state in Australia to get Cyberknife. This was really well received by so many people. Everyone thought it was a great idea and were only too happy to help out. I provided the contact details for the West Australian Premier and the Health Minister on this site. All the members of this new group had sent requests asking for Cyberknife to be installed at a hospital in West Australia. Initially they had replied with a sincere, if quite generic, response to most. It was heartwarming. I had approached politicians at federal and state level and many hadn't even replied. I had offered Perth the assistance of the team of doctors from USA which I spoke of earlier and that got a mention in the initial replies. However in early 2012 we got a reply from the Health Minister confirming that they would indeed be installing Australia's first Cyberknife. As you can imagine I was over the moon. People still responded that they wouldn't believe it until they actually saw Cyberknife in operation but I was happy with the response. A short while later a website link was sent to me. This was for the West Australian cancer centre and featured a page dedicated to Cyberknife and what it was all about. I attached this to my information pages and people began to believe. However about a week later the link to the Cyberknife information on the West Australian cancer centre's website no longer worked. The page still existed but the link was different. I attached the new link. In about a week this changed again. Now however there was no Cyberknife information on the website for the West Australian cancer centre. There was a page which had generic information on stereotactic radiotherapy and surgery but nothing specific about Cyberknife. I began to wonder what was happening. I contacted the Sir Charles Gardiner hospital which is where the West Australian cancer centre was based and asked them if indeed Cyberknife was being installed. They assured me it was. I just couldn't work out why the website had changed. The person I spoke with couldn't help with that query either.

A few weeks later I had still progressed no further in my investigations about the disappearing Cyberknife information. It was a mystery. However just as I was having some doubts I saw an advertisement in the employment section of a newspaper. It was an ad for the Sir Charles Gardiner hospital and they were looking for staff to work in the new cancer centre. They also pointed out the equipment the staff would be required to use. Cyberknife,

Australia's first, was one of the pieces of equipment that would be offered in this new centre. It mentioned that the facility would be operational in 2013 and listed some of the benefits of Cyberknife. One fact that amazed me and made me angry as well was that Australia's Gold Standard radiotherapy treatment at present was the Linear Accelerator. It also mentioned that Cyberknife was 100 times more powerful and seven times faster than what had been offered previously. Along with the versatility and accuracy of Cyberknife I wondered why it had taken so long to get Cyberknife to Australia.

I wouldn't say it was fanfare at this stage. But news within my network definitely spread quickly about Cyberknife finally coming to Australia. My friends in the UK made sure that I didn't take the foot off the pedal. The reminded me that this was one machine for over 20 million people. As, in the UK, they said that once we had one Cyberknife others should follow in other cities. My work was not done, however people who had watched my quest for several years were extremely happy. They mentioned that this was something concrete that people could see in the fight against cancer. All the money donated to cancer causes rarely showed such physical evidence of a way forward. One person contacted me that really showed that my fight had been worthwhile. Ashleigh Moore is an Order of Australia recipient. He is also chairman for cancer Voices South Australia. Ashleigh is also a senior leader with the Livestrong foundation which was set up by Lance Armstrong the famous or perhaps now infamous cyclist. Ashleigh contacted me to congratulate me on the hard work I had put in over the years. Ashleigh is also a cancer survivor. He had beaten head and neck cancer but was recently diagnosed with lung cancer. He was given few options but thought Cyberknife may be able to assist. He asked me for information on how to access Cyberknife but he also vowed to assist in getting more of these devices to Australian hospitals. As I had noticed in the past it is quite often not until people need it that they get on board to support raising awareness of Cyberknife. Ashleigh was now well and truly on board. I was delighted to have such a high profile supporter to work with.

Again the local media heard of this success. Star Fm, the local radio station wanted to do an interview. Mandy, the DJ was very vocal in her support of cancer causes. She had spoken to me several times before and wanted to share this latest news with the community. I was at the local McDonalds working with one of my clients when she rang, live on air. We spoke about the achievement of finally getting the Cyberknife to Australia. Mandy's on air co host was forced to leave work around this time due to a tumour behind the eye. This news was extremely relevant to her. It was the first interview of this kind. A positive one. I liked it.

NBN news also did a follow up of the progress. They had been very supportive from the early days at Lismore NBN. Georgie who had interviewed me many years ago was now working for Channel ten. She contacted me via Twitter to congratulate me. Then the most unexpected surprise of all. I got a huge certificate in the mail. It was an Australian of the year nomination. Well I was blown away. This was totally unexpected. It was not the reason I had done all of this but it was a very big surprise just before Christmas. Of course the television and radio stations wanted to do more stories on this latest development.

I could feel my identity changing. I had been the single dad struggling to keep his head above water and banging on about this strange cancer treatment. All of a sudden I was becoming respected within the community for someone who had shown determination and compassion towards a group of people in need and device that could assist many of them. Part of my work had been done but a lot more was still to be done.

# Chapter 35

# The Leah Chapman Cyberknife centre

A lovely lady I met several years ago, from the Gold Coast, was June. June had been diagnosed with an inoperable brain tumour. She was about 60 years of age at the time. She was about to enter the retirement years of her life with her husband. They were about to embark on a European trip. This diagnosis had changed everything. She began planning for her funeral. June was watching television one night. She had been feeling exceptionally depressed of late. June wondered why a country, considered the best in the world in cancer care, couldn't help her in her time of need. She saw the television program that I was on. She saw the story of Leah's brave fight and the discovery of this wonderful, state of the art cancer treatment. June wanted to know more.

June contacted me and asked if she could take up a small amount of my time. After hearing her story and realising how close she lived I invited her to have coffee and chat. She came down for the day and we met in Mullumbimby to see if I could be of assistance. Who would have thought that world class cancer care was being sourced in Mullumbimby! We had a lovely morning and I had as much information as I could pass on to June. She was in awe. She had been handed a death sentence but I was possibly assisting her in cheating death. All would be revealed. June returned to her home and set the wheels in motion. In only about a week she rang me to tell me that she was off to Malaysia for her treatment. I wished her luck and could sense the excitement in her voice.

Many people I had sent overseas I never heard from again. That wasn't the focus for me. I just hoped they were successful in being treated. However June did respond when she returned. She was amazed. June had one morning of treatment and spent the next few days shopping and siteseeing with her husband. It wasn't Europe but it was extremely rewarding.

We moved away from the area but I still keep in touch with June. She is still going strong and she got her trip to Europe. I was very happy for her and she has been a great supporter of me and Cyberknife. However she totally blew me away just recently. She asked me if I would mind if she started a quest to get the Cyberknife centre in Perth to be named the "Leah Chapman Cyberknife centre". Of course I was delighted. This is not a thing I had considered but it was a lovely tribute to the woman who had started all of this. It was also a nice way for June to give thanks to us all. June asked me for some photos and she set the rest up. The Facebook page with details is called - Please name Cyberknife centre in WA the "Leah Chapman Cyberknife centre".

# Chapter 36

# Some of the people we've met

Our lives, over a ten year period, had resembled a rollercoaster ride. Some amazing highs but unfortunately some very desperate lows. But during such times you can't help but encounter some amazing people. Some of these have been unexpected, some anonymous and some new and lifelong friends. A few are no longer with us and some have left great legacies. Leah met numerous wonderful people initially. Her initial diagnosis enabled us to meet some wonderful people who were helping out. Dr Jane knew people who assisted us when Leah needed it. She was an amazing source of knowledge as well as a great friend. She recommended Dr Nerene, who came to Leah's aid and performed Leah's initial surgery. Dr Rick was so compassionate. He was Leah's oncologist in Melbourne. All of our friends at that time were amazing and they still continue to be today. Many still send messages for Leah's birthday, the anniversary of her death or even our wedding anniversary. It's a true testament to friends who help out during a crisis but truly wonderful people continue that support years on. Leah also met many people throughout her treatments and her stay at the Gawler foundation. I still keep in contact with many of these people today. I am so happy that Leah was able to attend the Gawler retreat. It was a real highlight for her and I still refer to it today.

Jean, who Leah met in San Diego while getting the Gamma Knife treatment, was and still is truly amazing and a much loved part of our family. She has been such a generous lady and supplied such inspiration to Leah, myself and our children. She has been an angel for all of us.

Our time on Hamilton Island allowed us to meet some wonderful people and luckily, through mediums such as Facebook, we can keep in touch with these lovely friends on a regular basis. They actually had a memorial service for Leah after she passed away but we couldn't attend due to being away for Leah's funeral in Melbourne. This was held t the lovely little church on the island. They produced a video of the occasion which we still haven't been able to watch. But we met people through the kindy and the school. We met people through Leah's work at the resort and our positions in the HR department. We even made friends sitting by the pool or the beach. They have left us all with a lifetime of wonderful memories, support and friendship. I don't think I would have been able to cope with Leah's initial brain tumour diagnosis and treatment requirements anywhere else but Hamilton Island. We were meant to be there for a reason.

Once we moved to Wilsons Creek near Byron Bay we were blessed with such supportive and generous people within a wonderful community. Unfortunately, due to the enormity of the financial strain I was under, I didn't really get the chance to totally enjoy this environment fully. But I was so lucky the kids had the chance to experience it. Our neighbours, Terri, Paul, Jess and Finn were such amazing support for all of us. Terri had just lost her mum before we moved there and she and Leah clicked straight away. It would have been another great loss for her upon Leah's death and we used to talk of this on many occasions. But she and her family saved me so many times and we will all be eternally grateful for their support and friendship. Paul helped me set up the B&B, Leahbelles, gave me some wonderful lamps that he handmade and even a beautiful timber sculpture that filled a void on one of the walls.

When we first moved to the area we lived in a place called Rosebank. There we met Jacinta, Simon, Freyja and Bridie. They are a truly wonderful family and Leah and Jacinta also hit it off immediately. There weren't many people who Leah didn't get on wonderfully with. During Leah's final hospital stay Jacinta was amazing with her support of us all. She just took the kids under her wing and allowed us to try and help Leah as best we could. Since Leah's passing we have been lucky to maintain a great friendship which I hope will last forever.

The Wilsons Creek public school. Wow. What an amazing experience for Bim to enjoy. This gorgeous school in the rainforest, just a short trip from home, was a true blessing. The teachers, the principal and all the parents were just so supportive without even trying. I tried to help out at canteen, the odd working bee and activity days and this environment for Bim to spend five years of schooling was amazing. My little boy started there, Leah was lucky enough to see his first day. He developed skills and confidence in music, reading, art and many other facets of a well rounded education. He left a lovely and supportive group of friends when we were forced to relocate. But I hope we will stay in contact with them.

When Leah was heading off to Oklahoma for her Cyberknife treatment the editor of the local Lismore paper, Alex Easton, got wind of this and came and interviewed Leah. He followed up when she came back. He has done numerous articles since about our life since Leah's death. Many of our friends were so impressed by his pieces that my cousin's daughter actually wrote in to his paper and wrote a letter in memory of Leah. She lives in North Queensland but wanted to get the letter published in the paper that had supported Leah in her battle and now me in our ongoing challenges. Alex has even written an article since our move to the Central Coast. A follow up to let people know how we were going. Some of the media people I have met have been only interested in the short term. A story. Just one piece of the puzzle that has been our journey. But Alex has been extremely supportive and a pleasure to have known. I am sure he will write something about this little story in his paper.

Leah was determined to get the message out about these treatments that were commonplace overseas but we had to find out about by accident. Upon her return we did a bit of research. I stumbled across a story of a family in the UK. They didn't have the Cyberknife at the time but the husband, only in his thirties at the time, was not offered any help for his cancer. They were forced to the USA for treatment. They began a push to get Cyberknife in the UK. They started a foundation. They run a Cyberknife ball each year to raise funds and they began a Facebook group to gain support and raise awareness. This is where I got the idea for the Australian Facebook Cyberknife page. We have over 4000 supporters now. Alan was doing well and I get updates from Jan quite regularly. Unfortunately he did pass away recently and it was like I had lost a family member again. This was due to the support this family had shown me over the years. Cyberknife is sought after in the UK now. They have three hospitals offering it now due to people like Alan and Jan raising awareness. They have been truly inspirational. I was so inspired by their efforts that I wanted to replicate the activities they had undertaken. Alas my financial situation did not allow for this. I wanted to set up a charity just for Cyberknife as groups such as cancer councils don't promote equipment. I felt this was a huge gap in the cancer charity area. I wanted to fill that but had to do it in the manner that I could afford. It was a lot slower but it achieved results.

Sometimes the people are unknown but still leave an impression. I got a call from a friend. She asked if I could ring a man whose daughter was quite ill. She gave me his mobile number. I rang and the man told me the desperate story. He couldn't talk long as his daughter was in hospital and she was getting married in a few moments. She was sick from cancer and had just found out about Cyberknife but it appeared to be too late (again). He thanked me for the call but as she wouldn't be able to fly to access the treatment it was all a bit late. Her fiancé had wanted to show her how much he loved her so he asked her to marry him. I could relate to this desire. They were forced to have the wedding in the hospital. She died a few days later. They rang me to let me know. I had not met any of them and had only spoken for a few minutes but when I heard of the daughter's death I was devastated. I had tried to help many people in their quest for help, for information and for options. Some were successful, others not and some I never heard the result of. I hoped that they were successful. It didn't matter if I never heard the result as long as people were given options.


One story just touched many hearts straight away. This got a lot of exposure on all of my sites that had been set up. The situation was absolutely mind blowing. During the house raffle I conducted I gained a fair bit of media exposure and so did the Cyberknife. A young family from Sydney contacted me about their daughter Ila. Now Ila was two and a half years of age at the time. She had been diagnosed with a type of brain tumour. It was pretty serious so she was operated on at such a young age. It didn't really work as well as the parents had hoped. In fact a gland was damaged during the process which had some pretty severe ramifications. As well as the cancer she developed pretty severe side effects from the surgery. Her only choices now, in Australia, were really drastic chemo sessions that went for hours. Her mum contacted me about Cyberknife. I am not a doctor so couldn't help her immediately but I gave her the contact details of Leah's Cyberknife doctor in USA and some other valuable sources of information. The doctors in the USA requested scans and patient history of Ila and got back to her mum very promptly with the news that they thought they would be able to help Ila once she reached 3 years of age or so. However for them to access Cyberknife they would be required to travel overseas and due to the severity of Ila's condition air travel was not an option. This is one of the main reasons I have been so dedicated to getting the Cyberknife to Australia. If this is an option for people like Ila and they can't access it overseas then we needed to get it here quickly. For Ila, Cyberknife would need to be administered differently due to her lack of understanding the process involved with delivery of the treatment. In her case an anesthetic would need to be given and then the Cyberknife treatment could be used. The treatment plan would be different as well due to Ila's age but at least it was considered and option. All of this ended up being quite irrelevant in the end as the family would not be able to access this wonderful treatment. Ila's family have a marvelous site of inspiration and information on their brave little daughter:

**Keep Ila smilin' Fundraising and brain tumour awareness**

This is on Facebook and gives us hope that something can be done for this family and little Ila. I was asked by ABC radio to do a joint interview with Ila's dad. He explained the complexities of Ila's condition and I was asked about information on the Cyberknife. This was done in the hope it may have sparked some interest in the possibility of Ila having access to Cyberknife, which would in turn enable others to also access Cyberknife if it were brought to Australia to help this plucky little girl. Alas we are still waiting. I keep in contact with this family and like to keep up to date with Ila's progress. She is such a brave girl. She has a lot of support.

Denise Seymour is another lady I have had the privilege of getting to know. I have mentioned Denise before. She lost her son to Ostesarcoma a few years ago when he was only 17. She now has a foundation set up in Eriks memory.

Inspiration such as Denise's has taken me a long way on this journey, not just in writing this book, fighting for Cyberknife but also in day to day life. Leah had passion, strength and enthusiasm. She was motivated and determined. Upon her death I wanted to honour Leah by utilising those traits, after our initial time of grief and mourning, rather than allowing her death to render me useless. Denise has similar qualities and has achieved so much to honour the life her late son. Denise and Erik found out about Cyberknife too late, as do too many other Australians. The chances of Erik being able to be helped would have dramatically increased had they known about Cyberknife earlier.  This is frustrating and shattering for families. This is why we must get Cyberknife and some of the other treatment options, currently not available in Australia as soon as possible. Denise and her foundation are assisting with these endeavours. She is such a wonderful lady with great strength and a wonderful attitude even after what her family has been through. God bless her.

This is the link to her foundation:

http://erikhausoulsarcomafoundation.com/

Some of the others who I have been blessed to have met:

Many people I have met throughout this journey are in similar situations to me. Some are actually in much worse situations. I tried desperately to help Leah when the medical profession in Australia couldn't. We didn't quite make it. What might have been if we had earlier access to the options available overseas? I have found thousands of people in very similar situations. Leah was able to at least have a shot at beating this bloody awful disease. Many don't even get that opportunity. Most of the inspirational people I have met may have only featured in my life for a short time, even seconds but may have had a lasting impact. I met many people in hospital or doctors waiting rooms. Even shop keepers were supportive and helpful.

Many people, often from long distances, have come to my house for advice. Others have stopped me in the street for a chat or to poke a bit of fun at me. After all I have done a few bizarre things just to survive financially after the cancer roller coaster. But some people I never actually met at all but still had an impact on my life. Some contacts were just a letter or an email or a phone call that left an undeniable impression on me or Leah or the kids.

Here is one story of note that sticks in my mind. It happened when we just got back from Oklahoma. I received a phone call from a man in Sydney. He'd followed our story via the Byron Bay Echo online. He had just lost his wife and he said it wasn't from the cancer but due to the treatment she had received as a result of the cancer. She had been given radiation in Sydney and she never recovered. He is now concerned as the cancer is considered hereditary and he wishes to have better options for his children, already adults now, if they were to need it in the future. Of course he is hoping that they will not need anything at all. I have never met Bruce. But I communicate with him on a regular basis and we notify each other of breakthroughs in the medical field or even changes in our lives. We created an instant bond which resulted in an interest of Cyberknife. He has been an advocate for better choices for cancer patients in Australia. Cyberknife ticked all the boxes as far as he was concerned. We are both still waiting but feel closer to a result today than we did several years ago.

Another man I met through this quest is Jack, whose lovely wife was sick. She was looking forward to going overseas for Cyberknife. She needed to get a few things sorted here first. Some of her cancer could be treated here so they were focusing on getting that right first. Then she would go overseas to get treatment on the cancer that couldn't be treated in Australia. It was all a bit of a process and the last thing you need when dealing with cancer. They were a lovely couple and I got quite involved and also excited about the prospects. However Jack's angel never made it. She never got to go overseas for Cyberknife and Jack was a shattered man. I must say so was I. I got to know some of these people. Many of these outcomes hurt me nearly as much as the families concerned. This was another extremely frustrating situation for everyone concerned. It turned into absolute devastation with the outcome which could have been quite different had we been able to offer Cyberknife in Australia. Jack and I still chat from time to time even though, again, we've never met. I would have loved to have met Claire. She had great support in Jack but she just couldn't make it. This has been an all too familiar story.

Another source of inspiration for me was from a Melbourne woman named Samantha Lehman. She lost her brother to cancer and started the Warwick foundation in his memory to help young adults with cancer. She does a wonderful job and the manner in which she does it is very admirable. She creates lots of fun events that attract huge amounts of interest and generate lots of donations and awareness.

http://www.thewarwickfoundation.org.au

Ceridwen is another lady who contacted me on behalf of her mum who was sick with cancer. We were still at Wilsons Creek when she rang and it turned out she lived on the Central Coast. She seemed a very passionate and driven woman. I gave her what information she needed while I was still at our home in Wilsons Creek. I then caught up with her when we moved to the Central Coast. She had heard of our story and wanted to help but also needed information on the treatment for her mother. Unfortunately her mum died a few days later after Ceridwen and I met for the first time. They became aware of me when they met another lady, Josie, who had lung cancer and actually had Cyberknife in Malaysia. Josie had stayed with us in my bed and breakfast some time earlier. Ceridwen has such energy and drive and is also keen to assist with getting

Cyberknife to Australia. This was unfortunately another story with an unhappy ending.

Kelly Delaney is another from the UK. Her father could have been assisted by Cyberknife but they couldn't access it due to the cost of it in UK. One centre was set up due to generous private donations so the Cyberknife could be utilised by NHS patients. But the government was taking it's time approving this. It's these delays that can make the difference between life and death. Kelly is one of the many campaigning to change things in the UK. She and the others initiating the fight for Cyberknife in the UK have really made a difference. It is amazing what strength you gain when a loved one needs your help. They now have five hospitals offering Cyberknife in the UK and she wanted one of these to offer Cyberknife through the NHS. She was using many different avenues to make herself heard, not just for her dad but for others in similar situations in the UK. However while all this was happening, Kelly's younger sister was diagnosed with cancer and passed away quite quickly and suddenly. Life can be cruel some times. As I said, this book is our story, which I find quite bizarre but everyone has a story to tell. Many of them unfortunately have sad endings. The shock of Tammy's passing had an immediate effect on all of us who had been supporting Kelly with her quest. We still celebrate Tammy's life and help each other when birthdays or an anniversary comes around. Through Cyberknife many unique friendships have formed and we all have a common bond. I think this is about the only consolation that comes out of all of this cancer stuff. Imagine the lives that could have been changed if these people were able to access it more readily.

A brilliant lady I met throughout my quest was Ruth Peberdy. She was another from the UK petitioning successfully to get Cyberknife there. She lost her husband several years ago after a battle with pancreatic cancer. They found out about Cyberknife in Florida and Ron became the UK's first Cyberknife patient. As Ruth came from a medical background she saw the benefit of having access to this technology. She did lots of petitioning and fundraising and in a few short years the UK now has the five centres offering Cyberknife with more on the way. She has had many news articles written about her determination and I actually feature in one. I feel honoured to be associated with such a knowledgeable and successful woman. Ruth has also generated numerous substantial donations which have helped to ensure her success. One of these donations was in the form of millions of pounds from an anonymous donour. This was a brilliant and deserved reward for all her hard work. If I didn't see other success stories I don't think I could have mustered the energy to continue with all of this as long as I have. Ruth has an organisation set up in her late husband's name and is a wonderful source of information. This is the website she started to assist in her endeavours.

www.cyber-ron.com

Many other wonderful people have assisted and inspired me over the years. Terry is the minister from Hamilton Island and was our neighbor. He is truly a great friend to us all. What an amazing man. Terry was so supportive of me over many years. He took me aside as an individual and showed genuine friendship while offering much needed support. He is a great role model for any male in today's society. Terry took an active interest in our entire family but was very mindful of each of us as individuals. I have extremely fond memories of the friendship offered by Terry while we were on Hamilton Island and since.

Colleen, who I spoke of earlier, deserves recognition as well. She helped her friend get Cyberknife in Malaysia. We had spoken heaps about getting the word out but it always fell on deaf ears. Colleen lives on the Gold Coast and one afternoon visited the Tibetan monks who were visiting the Byron region. She popped into see me for a cup of tea on the way home to the Gold Coast. Where we lived at the time is not a place you just pop in to visit. It was a planned trip. But Colleen did it. We met for the first time after knowing each other for numerous years. It was such a lovely and unexpected meeting and amazing to finally meet such a wonderful woman. Her friend is still doing well and I get updates from Colleen and her family and friends quite often. It would have been comforting to have a friend such as Colleen assist you at such an important time as when her friend went to Malaysia for Cyberknife. I know how her friend would have felt and I know she would have appreciated having support while undergoing cancer treatment.

Helen Robertson is another who fought a brave battle but sadly lost. She was keen to access Cyberknife for her cancer but time beat her. Her daughter got married a short time after we met and Helen was able to attend the wedding which is comforting. Helen made sure the government knew they were letting people down by not getting better choices to Australia for cancer patients. She has had many questions brought up in parliament. She may have left us just after her daughter's wedding but she definitely left her legacy. I feel an obligation to carry on with that.

Amanda Ryall has also helped so much. We have never met but she gave me support and guidance through some tough times. She was very supportive early on in the Cyberknife quest when my grief was quite pronounced after Leah's death. To assist in writing to politicians she drafted a brilliant letter for supporters to send off. Amanda emailed it to me for approval and I cried when I read it. I guess that was the approval she was after. It's on the Facebook site so people can individualise it and send it on. Amanda and her husband live in Japan. Japan has about 20 hospitals with Cyberknife. The Victorian government actually did a study tour of the Cyberknife centres in Japan in 2010. They then committed $8 million to a cancer centre featuring

Cyberknife but were ousted in the State election later in the year. The incoming government decided not to go ahead with the idea of bringing Cyberknife to Australia.

Others in need of mention here are all of the staff as well as Leah's wonderful friends at the Gawler foundation. Anita and Byron who are the children's God parents. All of our friends from Melbourne, Hamilton Island and the Byron region. I must also thank all of our other family and friends who assisted so much throughout the entire journey.

I must mention Cath who had joined Leah and I in India on our journey for a miracle. Leah had known Cath for many years and got to know her about 10 or 12 years ago. Her entire family are such down to earth and generous friends. It was a great pleasure to have travelled to India with her. The memories of that trip are quite special and Cath played a big part in that. However just after I moved to the Central Coast I got a call from Pauline in Melbourne. Cath had suffered a huge aneurism and passed away suddenly. No signs no symptoms. I was devastated. So to was the family. This indeed was a tragedy. Cath was about my age so it got me thinking some more.

Obviously there are many more people who had or still have a great impact on our lives. This happens to everyone. It just seems that due to our experiences it may happen a bit more often. I don't mind as I gain more inspiration from new experiences and the people involved. I must thank everyone who has helped us along our journey. No matter how small a part you have played you have had an influence. Even the negative ones have helped shape our future. But I do prefer to dwell on and remember fondly the wonderful people and experiences we have had even during some of our darkest times.

# One special thank you

Through all of this, one special person has kept me sane. After Leah died he would often cry himself to sleep. He had never known Leah to be constantly healthy but they loved and adored each other. I still find little notes around the house, from Leah to Bim, telling him how much she loves him. After Leah's death Bim was like a rock to me and he was only six years old. He loved his surroundings, had amazing friends and support. He loved his school and sports and he really showed appreciation, in many ways, of my effort to save our home and lifestyle. He took nothing for granted. How could I not try and save our home from the banks with such lovely children around me. Bim would often answer the phone when the banks called, sometimes he'd say I wasn't available to save me the agony of dealing with them again and again. If I was upset he would comfort me. He loves hugs. He loves kisses and adversity drove us closer together. Friends often said that Leah would have passed comforted by the idea that the children had me. It's a huge responsibility. Both the children had totally different ways of evolving after Leah's death. Rebecca sought solitude and Bim sought strength from the family. If I was short of money Bim would go to his piggy bank. He helped with the B&B and the guests loved it. I received a letter from a previous guest, after my news of Leahbelles sale, from a lovely couple who mentioned Bim in their thoughts and had lovely memories of meeting him. He has that effect on people. When all avenues were exhausted and we were forced from our home, friends and security, Bim was so willing to help with the move to our new life and make it work. He went to a new school with over 700 kids after being at a school all his life with just 50. This was extremely difficult for him. I could see it in his eyes. He never complained. He always had a smile or a joke. He has made the transition now and even has a trip back to the Byron region for occasional holidays to stay with our close friends next door to our old home. The change in him has been monumental. He plays numerous sports. He won an Academic Excellence award at his primary school. He was one of eight from the 700 who were selected. Imagine how proud I was. This was a regional award so he was presented with it at a ceremony featuring schools and students from all over the area. He helps around the house. He makes his bed each day, does the dishes and cleans up around home. As I said, he knows the effort we put in and he gets the rewards. His school work is organised and amazing. His new teachers love him. People have said for ages that he is mature beyond his years. I could not be more proud of my little man. Bim has now started High school. He continues to achieve high results. He got many excellence awards in his first year and now attends a school with 1200 students. What a change he has gone through. He went without for years and we are still not totally back on our feet but he is now appreciating the effort we are putting in to make a new beginning. I owe him so much. I cannot thank him enough for his tolerance, love and support. I couldn't ask for a better son. Thank you Bim. I love you.

## Also, a huge thank you, to you

Thank you so much for buying this book. People said to me, once they'd gotten to know me, that they only knew certain aspects of our journey. They felt we'd had an interesting time with things and that I should fill in the gaps. This I have done. Even if you didn't feel like reading it and just jumped to the back then you have still assisted in the goal of bringing better and more cancer treatment options to Australia. Leah once said, as I have also mentioned several times since, that if we could save one life, spare one family from going through what we were forced to, then it would be worth it. I know of many who have gone overseas to receive Cyberknife and now lead full and healthy lives. My battle has been worth it for them. The fact that we now have information about Cyberknife, which we didn't have just five short years ago, is a major step forward. This information also assists patients and families take control of their own treatment. They can research other options and make a decision as to which one is best for them, even if they are all only available overseas.

However my quest is not complete. People who cannot travel or cannot afford to travel are being disadvantaged with these treatments only being available overseas. That's why I have written this story, as it's the only way I could see to raise the money to get Cyberknife to Australia.

Thanks again for your support.

14694989R00168

Printed in Great Britain
by Amazon.co.uk, Ltd.,
Marston Gate.